Roz Shapiro
_,11/88

You are what a
Vector looks like and
acts like

Lve

FROM
VICTIM
TO
VICTOR

FROM
VICTIM
TO
VICTOR

The
Wellness Community Guide
to Fighting for Recovery
for Cancer Patients
and Their Families

Harold H. Benjamin, Ph.D.
with Richard Trubo

Foreword by Richard Steckel, M.D.
Director of the Jonsson Comprehensive Cancer Center, UCLA

JEREMY P. TARCHER, INC.
Los Angeles

Distributed by St. Martin's Press
New York

Library of Congress Cataloging in Publication Data

Benjamin, Harold H.
   From victim to victor.

   Bibliography.
   Includes index.
   1. Cancer—Psychological aspects.   2. Cancer—Psychosomatic as-
pects.   I. Trubo, Richard.   II. Title.
RC262.B36   1987   616.99'40651   87-10157
ISBN 0-87477-452-7

Jeremy P. Tarcher, Inc.
9110 Sunset Blvd.
Los Angeles, CA 90069

Design by Rosa Schuth

Manufactured in the United States of America
10   9   8   7   6   5   4   3   2   1

First Edition

CONTENTS

PART I: INFORMATION ABOUT CANCER

How does cancer start?   What is the difference between a benign and malignant tumor?   What is the immune system?   What is the "surveillance theory"? Can stress affect the development of cancer?   What is the "fight-or-flight response" and does it have an effect on the development of or the recovery from cancer?

Can a predisposition to cancer be inherited?   Can environment play a part in the development of cancer?   Can my beliefs and behavior have an effect on the development of cancer?

What is biofeedback?

Can a traumatic event I experienced before the diagnosis have an effect on my recovery?   How can I change my emotional reactions to help my fight for recovery?

PART II: DEALING WITH REACTIONS TO CANCER

PART III: BEING A PATIENT ACTIVE

PART IV: INTIMACY

PART V: CONFRONTING CONFUSING ISSUES

PART VI: FAMILY AND FRIENDS ASK

PART VII: ABOUT THE WELLNESS COMMUNITY

They have led us with knowledge and understanding:

ACKNOWLEDGMENT AND DEDICATION

I acknowledge the importance of and dedicate this book to:

- The thousands of people with cancer who have permitted me to be a part of their lives and learn from them how important each day is, that every question has an answer and that every problem has a solution.

- Harriet Benjamin, whose support, understanding, and encouragement made all this possible.

- Charles E. (Chuck) Dederich and Harold Stone, Ph.D. who, while we were together, unselfishly shared with me their wisdom and insight, which form the underpinnings of The Wellness Community.

- Norman Cousins, who said exactly the right thing at exactly the right time.

- The professional staff of The Wellness Community, all of whom were and are a part of the evolution of a concept that may have an effect on the world: Shannon Behrens McGowan, M.A., M.F.C.C.; Florence Porter, B.A.; Janet Smith, Ph.D., M.F.C.C.; Celeste Torrens, L.C.S.W., M.F.C.C.; Joan Ellen Caine, M.A., M.F.C.C.; Joanna Bull, M.A., M.F.C.C.; Lynne Weingarten, M.A., M.F.C.C.; Allen Berkowitz, Ph.D.; Mitch Golant, Ph.D.

- Celeste Torrens, who saw to it that I didn't make too many mistakes, and Diane Josephs, who did much of the nuts-and-bolts work.

- Howard P. Ladd, chairman of the board of The Wellness Community, and board members Basil Anderman, Neal Bermas, Gerald Bronstein, Douglas K. Freeman, George Green, Richard Gunther, Lynette Kurtzman, William Minkin, Rose Rashmir, Carl Rheuban, Norma Ring, and Seth Weingarten.

FOREWORD

Harold Benjamin is a special man who has had a highly successful career as a lawyer, social psychologist, community leader and activist, administrator, and philanthropist. Most recently, he has devoted his time and efforts to The Wellness Community, a program he founded in Santa Monica, California, that provides free psychological and emotional support to cancer patients. As director of that program, he has accumulated enormous experience in addressing the psychosocial needs of people with cancer. In *From Victim to Victor* he draws on that experience to examine many of the questions that plague cancer patients.

Dr. Benjamin's book brings into sharp relief the various meanings of the word "patient." As a noun, *patient* refers to a person with a malady who is being cared for by a professional; as an adjective, *patient* describes a person who is complacent, passive, or long-suffering. It has long appeared to me that, for all but a few of us, *patient* frequently carries both of those meanings in whatever context it is used.

But Dr. Benjamin explodes the myth that an individual with cancer must accept passively whatever fate has in store and reminds us that there is much that can be done to actively maintain or reestablish physical well-being. He points out to cancer patients the pitfalls that can further complicate an already serious situation, and suggests methods of avoiding or minimizing these dangers. He also encourages practicing many positive techniques he has observed cancer patients using in their fight for recovery.

I have yet to meet a physician who would not prefer to relate to his or her cancer patient as a partner in the fight for recovery. Clearly, the methods suggested in this book can strengthen such a partnership. In fact, many physicians from our Comprehensive Cancer Center at UCLA support their patients' desire to take a more active role in enhancing the quality of their lives and perhaps improving their chances of recovery by referring them to The Wellness Community.

Throughout this book, Dr. Benjamin makes it clear that techniques such as guided imagery and group interaction can support and enhance good medical care but are not substitutes for such professional treatment. While he encourages patients to take more active responsibility in their fight for recovery, he is also sensitive to the tendency of patients to "blame" themselves for acquiring or failing to conquer the illness and stresses that there is absolutely *no* justification for assuming such blame.

In the same vein, while it is well accepted that attitudes and feelings can be positive, life-enhancing forces in an individual's battle against cancer, Dr. Benjamin reminds us that this is not equivalent to saying that emotions "cause" cancer or that bad thoughts or feelings are responsible for a person's failure to recover from the disease. Though the scientific community now acknowledges that the mind and body are a continuum, "biology" *cannot* always be controlled with the methods currently available to medicine. To suggest otherwise is all too common among some individuals who advocate "alternative therapy" as a replacement for good medical treatment, a position Dr. Benjamin assuredly does not share.

Ultimately, it is clear that there is no single method or universal technique for taking a more active role in the cancer-recovery process. But the important principle for cancer patients to grasp is that they have the option of participating in this process. I know of no other book that makes this point more cogently or blends so well both emotional support and practical advice than does *From Victim to Victor.* Harold Ben-

jamin speaks to us directly from his experience with the
thousands of cancer patients who have chosen to be Patients
Active in their fight for recovery.

RICHARD J. STECKEL, M.D.
Director, Jonsson Comprehensive Cancer Center
University of California, Los Angeles (UCLA)

PREFACE

This book is about cancer. But it's not about coping with cancer, learning to live with it, making the best of it, or dying from it. It is about living, fighting to recover, *and, if possible, recovering.* It's about participating in the fight for recovery—being a Patient Active instead of a passive, hopeless, helpless victim of the illness. It's about hope ... always hope. Not false hope, but a realistic appraisal of the future based on something other than the myths and fables that surround cancer. In essence, it's about the conversion from victim to Victor.

While directed at individuals with cancer, *From Victim to Victor* will also help friends and family deal with cancer patients in a more enlightened way, much to the benefit of all parties. It is also designed to teach healthy individuals to contemplate the possibility of cancer from a more realistic, and therefore less horrifying, perspective. In the process, they may learn to alter their lives in ways that make their chances of developing cancer a little more remote.

In my research, I have observed and consulted the true experts in the field—cancer patients, several thousand of them. All of them have actively participated in their fight for recovery at The Wellness Community, a cost-free program for people with cancer in Santa Monica, California, of which I am founder and executive director. Much of the material in this book is based on the experiences of these patients.

You will read about The Wellness Community throughout this book, because the Patient Active concept was developed here. But understand that I use The Wellness Community only for purposes of illustration. You do not need a Wellness Community to use the Patient Active concept in your own fight for recovery. You can use it wherever you are and whatever your circumstances. You can use it alone or with others, continuously or sporadically. Whether you use every suggestion or just one, you can only benefit by doing so.

In this book, cancer patients will learn how to join with their physicians in actively participating in their fight for recovery—that is, how to be Patients Active. As you read along, you will see that our fundamental philosophy, developed during years of interaction with cancer patients, is that *cancer patients who participate in their fight for recovery along with their physicians—instead of acting as hopeless, helpless, passive victims of the illness—will improve the quality of their lives and just may enhance the possibility of their recovery.* (Because this statement reflects the foundation of the Patient Active concept, variations of it appear throughout the book.)

While no one as yet knows with certainty whether such participation actually enhances the recovery process, it does improve the quality of life. I have seen this occur time and again over my ten years of observing thousands of people with cancer.

Integral to the Patient Active concept is an understanding of the word *Victor.* A Victor, as we define it at The Wellness Community, is a person who has been diagnosed as having cancer and has taken back some control in his life, has become a Patient Active, and considers himself a Victor, no matter what his physical condition. If you have cancer, you can transform yourself from victim to Victor by a change of attitude. This alters the entire context in which you live your life and may enhance the possibility of recovery.

Both The Wellness Community and this book are intended to be adjuncts to conventional medical treatment. Neither offers an alternative to traditional care. Although we do not require our participants at The Wellness Community to be in the care of a conventional physician, less than 1 percent forgo conventional medical treatment. We firmly believe that the primary treatment for cancer is provided by the medical profession, and we encourage compliance with your physician's advice. As James J. Strain, M.D., reported at the American Cancer Society conference on "Human Values and Cancer" in 1987, noncompliance can make the possibility of recovery more remote.

In this book, I will not consider the medical or spiritual aspects of cancer treatment. Certainly the physical, spiritual, and mental aspects of life cannot be completely separated, and all three are integral parts of total cancer patient care. But medical and spiritual matters are best left to the experts in those fields. This book will concern itself only with the mind—the psychological, emotional, social, and philosophical.

There is no question that a great need exists for the kind of psychosocial support for cancer patients outlined in this book. Forty or fifty years ago, those who developed cancer were treated either medically or surgically. Too often, the results were unfortunate—and exactly as expected. Life expectancy after the diagnosis was usually short, and there wasn't anything the patient could do.

But that's no longer true. Because of medical progress, many cancer patients now recover completely, and many others live for long periods of time. In the process, cancer changes them profoundly. They need support and new ways of thinking to adjust to those changes. In addition, without social and psychological support, they find themselves in limbo, perceived by themselves and by others as modern-day lepers. They are unjustly ashamed and embarrassed by their disease.

That's where social, psychological, and emotional support comes in. Since The Wellness Community opened in 1982, it has helped thousands of cancer patients and is still growing dramatically. People who have devoted their lives to helping cancer patients, including many prominent oncologists and psychologists, serve on the professional advisory board. Norman Cousins is honorary chairman of the board of directors. Most of the participants come on the recommendation of their physicians. Thus, The Wellness Community concept of the Patient Active is not just a theory of a small group of people but is supported and encouraged by highly respected health-care providers. Every aspect of our program is based on scientific fact or reasonable scientific hypothesis. The emerging field studying the effect emotions have on physical well-being is known as psychoneuroimmunology. In many professional circles, the Community is considered an integral and reliable part of total cancer patient care and an adjunct to conventional medical treatment. (For additional information about The Wellness Community and how it evolved, see chapter 54.)

The most important word in the name is *Community*, signifying the underlying principle of everything we do— namely, making it possible for each participant to build a support group. It is my hope that this book will serve as a "support group within covers" for you, wherever you are and whatever your circumstances.

1. Beginning the fight for recovery

In this book, you will meet many Patients Active who have agreed to share their stories. They will tell you how they actively participated in their fight for recovery and how you, if you have cancer, can be active in yours.

In converting from patient passive to Patient Active and from victim to Victor, you'll join the ranks of people like Steven, who was diagnosed as having lymphoma several years ago. In one of The Wellness Community's Sharing Groups (the forum where most patients are introduced to the program), Steven told the newcomers that even though he had a loving and supportive wife and many good and empathic friends, he needed more:

> I hope we all have supportive families and friends, but even the best of friends can't begin to appreciate what we cancer patients experience. My best friend—even my brother—can't be expected to understand what I'm going through as well as Susan does or Janice [two other cancer patients]. The help and encouragement you get from other cancer patients are absolutely unique.

Like most people, Steven had made all his own decisions before his illness. He had been independent and had spent much of his time helping others. However, cancer changed him. He was no longer the successful radio, television, and political expert. He had become, in his own mind, only a "cancer patient"—nothing more.

When Steven first heard his diagnosis, he was depressed and despondent, believing he was doomed to a short, unpleasant future without friends or joy. He felt completely without control over his life. More important, cancer became his entire reality. Like many others, he couldn't bring himself to say the word. He called it the "Big C."

But when Steven learned there were actions he could take to fight for his recovery, he was filled with hope and expectations that he could once again know joy and friendship and regain control of his life. He realized that cancer was only a part of him. He met others who talked about cancer as a fact of life, not as the curse of a slow, torturous death starting from the moment of diagnosis. To them, cancer was a burden to be borne and dealt with, not an inescapable punishment visited on them by a vengeful and unfair fate. He spent time with others who had once been where he was and who now were living happy, productive lives.

Recovery was possible, Steven saw. Not promised, not guaranteed...but possible. "Because we are with other cancer patients, including some who have recovered, we know that we don't have to be passive," Steven said. "We know that it's possible for every one of us to participate in our own fight for our recovery, and to work at it. And that work can certainly bring about more happiness and may help us recover."

You won't find answers in this book. You will find suggestions and questions to help you see what alternatives you have and which are best for you. Don't view the statement "it's all up to you" as a burden, but as a reminder of your freedom, right, and ability to make whatever decisions you believe to be in your best interest.

As you read this book, it's important to understand that everything you are doing and decide to do in the future about the illness is right for you. You know more about you and your needs than any other person can possibly know. At any given moment, you are doing what you feel is best for you; despite what anyone else thinks or says, you're right.

Because I want this book to have the same positive effect on people with cancer, wherever they are, that a Sharing Group has on individuals new to The Wellness Community, let me describe such a group briefly. There are no professionals in Sharing Groups, only cancer patients, their families, and friends—and Victors.

At a Sharing Group, each Victor and (with very few exceptions) each newcomer tells his or her story. There is always an enormous amount of energy, good will, friendship, and laughter in the room—and sometimes tears. But it's seldom depressing.

Most people have never before had a chance to talk about their cancer to anyone who wasn't shocked or scared by the word or who didn't respond in hushed, anxious tones. They have felt ostracized, alone, ashamed, beaten down, depressed, and, worst of all, helpless. They have believed they had no alternative but to relinquish their entire lives and volition to others.

But at a Sharing Group, they hear people speak about cancer in the same way they discuss any other very unpleasant experience—not with awe and superstition, but with candor and reality. They realize instantly that not everyone diagnosed with cancer dies from it; they see vital, vibrant, involved, interesting, charismatic people living full and complete lives, who—at one time or another—have been in the same situation they are in. And they recognize that recovery is a possibility for them, too, thus restoring hope and the will to live. At the same time, their own feelings of shame, guilt, and embarrassment over having cancer are relieved because none of the others with whom they're sitting seems ashamed or embarrassed about having cancer.

Many of the newcomers—like many of you—will ultimately become Victors. Many of these Victors have been symptom-free for years, and all believe they played an important part in their own recovery. One of the Victors in almost every Sharing Group is Flo Porter, a vivacious, perky, attractive 46-year-old woman. Of all the people with cancer I know, no one has worked harder to recover.

In 1979, Flo had her second mastectomy, followed by chemotherapy. She immediately became involved in telling her story to other cancer patients, hoping to be of as much help to them as she could. She went back to school, altered her attitudes about her parents and children, joined a mastectomy self-help group at her local Y, and became active in helping single women deal with the specific issues of dating after a mastectomy. She also had reconstructive surgery and supported other women about to undergo the same procedure. She has been symptom-free since the second mastectomy.

Another Victor is Al Fractor, a trim, athletic, gravelly-voiced retired lithographer who is one of the most candid men I've ever met. In 1981, at age 61, he had colon cancer. Immediately after surgery, he involved himself in personal efforts to get well, along with the fine medical treatment he was receiving. He joined a therapy group and began studying nutrition. He made significant life changes, including retiring from his occupation. He became a proponent of taking control of one's life. Al has been symptom-free since early 1982 and leads an extremely active life.

Flo and Al used the distilled wisdom of many other cancer patients in their fight for recovery, and you can, too. Recently I asked a group of participants what general advice they would give to a cancer patient who wanted to change from a victim to a Victor, from a patient passive to a Patient Active. These are their answers, all of which will be discussed in detail later in this book:

- Be aware that the diagnosis of cancer is not necessarily a sentence of death. There are millions of people in the United States to whom cancer is now a memory.

- Be aware that there's always the possibility of joy and involvement in life.

- Be aware that you did not cause your cancer.

- Be aware that you are not to blame if the course of the illness does not go as you want it to.

- Follow the advice of your physician or other healing professional.

- Form a partnership with your physician or other healing professional, rather than an employer/employee relationship (with you as the employee).

- Know that you are not helpless and that you can be the most important member of the team fighting for recovery.

- Take all reasonable steps to maintain social contacts at least as extensively as you did before the diagnosis.

- Retain as much control of your life as is reasonable. Start by taking control of your eating and exercise habits.

- Spend a reasonable amount of time with other cancer patients.

- Learn as much about your illness as you consider appropriate.

- Keep your stress levels as low as possible.

- Take an inventory of the way you react to life events to see if you are responding in ways that may not be in your best interest. In particular, consider whether you repress anger and whether you are strongly attached to someone or something that has been lost.

- Learn to meditate and practice your own guided imagery.

- Be aware that cancer is not a curse, nor is it shameful; it is only a disease like any other disease.

- Maintain hope for recovery and whatever else you want from life.

- Talk to friends and family and tell them what you want from them; ask them what they want from you.

At this point, some of the above suggestions may seem too vague to understand completely. Some may even seem frivolous or impossible to accomplish. But as we look at these areas in more detail, you will learn why so many other cancer patients believe them to be important.

So that you can begin to use this book in the way best for you, let me explain the format. Following are 54 short chapters, each built around questions that cancer patients frequently ask about dealing with and overcoming cancer. Over the past ten years, patients at The Wellness Community have asked these questions over and over again, not only of me, but also of physicians, psychologists, other cancer patients, and anyone else who will listen.

From conversations with cancer patients, physicians, and psychologists, I have culled those questions that come up most often. The answers in this book are composites based on the experiences of hundreds of cancer patients.

The question-and-answer format is used here for two reasons. First, many cancer patients feel relieved just to learn that their questions are no different from those of others. Second, the answers will reduce stress, because you will find that the facts are never as discouraging or as anxiety-producing as what you imagine.

The earlier chapters are concerned with more technical material that provides the foundation for the suggestions and observations that follow. But you don't have to read the chapters in sequence for the book to be meaningful. Because you may choose to read a later chapter before those that precede it, some of the information is set forth in more than one chapter.

Now that you know something about The Wellness Community, what a Sharing Group is, and why this book is being written, try to imagine yourself in a lovely old yellow house, in a living room filled with large chairs and overstuffed couches. You are with fifteen or twenty other people in a Sharing Group. I hope you will react to this book as our participants do to Sharing Groups—with renewed hope, a strong will to live, and replenished energy—with the belief and hope that your own activities can have a beneficial effect on your recovery process and will improve the quality of your life. So let's move forward together.

I
INFORMATION ABOUT CANCER

2. What exactly is cancer?

છ

Most people visualize the onset of cancer as the emergence of a powerful, invincible cancer cell that will grow larger and larger until it kills us. We also assume that this dreaded cell appears only in the bodies of people who eventually develop the illness.

But the cancer cell is *not* an all-powerful, destructive, invincible force; rather, it is a weak, erratic, and confused cell, and all of us have such cells proliferating in our bodies at various times. In the great majority of cases, when a cancer cell comes into being, it is attacked and destroyed by our immune system before it can do any harm, and we don't develop cancer. But, as you will see, when cancer cells appear and the immune system fails to do its job, the result is cancer.

NORMAL AND ABNORMAL CELLS

The human body is a collection of cells that perform separate specific functions, each linked to the others and operating in a highly regulated manner. All normal cells have internal controls that determine when they start and stop performing their functions. In this cycle, a normal cell is born, matures and performs its designated function, and then dies, and a new cell replaces it.

When new cells are required, the existing ones divide in two, and those two divide again and so on until the exact number of required new cells is achieved. Under normal circumstances, the birth and death of a cell is an exquisitely precise process. But if a cell fails to stop dividing when it is supposed to or fails to die on schedule, many problems arise.

Cancer is perhaps the most serious problem caused by this cellular malfunction. Cancer results when, for reasons still unknown, a normal cell divides and gives birth to an abnormal cell that does not respond to normal regulation—that is, it continues to divide after the need for replacement cells is met, and it refuses to die on schedule. If unchecked, such cells divide and subdivide without end and eventually join together to form a clump of cells—a tumor. As the tumor becomes larger, it impedes the functioning of nearby organs by intruding on their space and by interfering with their supply of oxygen and nutrients. Eventually the healthy organs are destroyed.

Tumors can be of two types, benign or malignant. A *benign* tumor, while often serious in nature, may cause problems exclusively at its place of origin. It can usually be excised from the body by surgery, thus putting the problem to rest.

By contrast, a *malignant* tumor cell has the capacity to travel to other parts of the body in a process called metastasis. Normal cells are picky about where they will grow: a clump of normal liver cells accidentally transferred to a leg muscle will not grow there but will die and become absorbed by the surrounding tissue. Malignant cells, on the other hand, may thrive in their new environment, growing to form a large tumor and causing the same type of problems in the new location they caused at the original site. *Cancer* is the generic name for over one hundred diseases that share the general characteristics of malignant cells described above.

THE IMMUNE SYSTEM: OUR FIRST LINE OF DEFENSE

Our immune system is an intricate system designed to protect the body from disease and from "foreigners" that invade through a break in the skin, via food or other ingested matter, or by way of the air we breathe or the rays to which we are exposed. We have all become aware of just how important the immune system is since the advent of AIDS (acquired immune deficiency syndrome); the AIDS patient eventually succumbs to a disease (such as pneumonia) from which he would have been protected were it not for his severely impaired immune system.

From the cancer patient's point of view, the immune system's most important function is to destroy cancer cells as they appear or after they have formed a tumor. Motion pictures have actually shown cancer cells being attacked and destroyed by the cells of the immune system. It's an inspiring sight. Some cancer patients cheer when they see it.

The power of the immune system is particularly apparent when it rejects transplanted vital organs such as kidneys and hearts. When the new organ is placed in the body, the immune system may recognize it as foreign and do everything in its power to reject it. For that reason, before a transplant that is not from an identical twin can have any chance of success, the immune system must be suppressed by drugs. (On the dark side, however, the transplant recipient is rendered more vulnerable to other diseases while his or her immune system is depressed.)

One way to think about cancer is not that the cancer cell is strong, but that the body's immune system is not strong enough to carry out its assigned, normal function of removing cancer cells from the body. This view of cancer is generally known as the immune surveillance theory.

STRESS DEPRESSES THE IMMUNE SYSTEM

The body's automatic reaction to becoming aware of an event that is perceived as unpleasant is called the "fight or flight" response. It is this response that weakens the immune system. Now that we know a robust immune system is one of the keys to cancer prevention and may have a beneficial effect on the possibility of recovery from cancer, the subject of stress becomes extremely important, because it is a well-established fact that when we undergo most types of prolonged, unremitting, negative stress our immune systems become depressed. That fact has been firmly established by thousands of studies; the Institute for the Advancement of Health has published a two-volume compendium that includes summaries of 2,316 of them. (Although the link between stress and illness itself has not been proven to everyone's satisfaction, it has received enough attention to merit serious consideration.)

The following chart (Figure 2-1) represents the chain of events that results in the immune system–depressing fight-or-flight response:

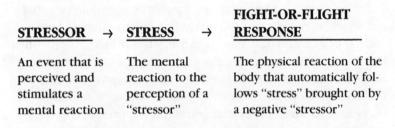

STRESSOR →	STRESS →	FIGHT-OR-FLIGHT RESPONSE
An event that is perceived and stimulates a mental reaction	The mental reaction to the perception of a "stressor"	The physical reaction of the body that automatically follows "stress" brought on by a negative "stressor"

Figure 2-1. The stress chain of events.

Stressor and Stress   If you are walking down the street and observe a car passing, that event is not a stressor, since it does not evoke a mental reaction. Suppose, however, that you recognize a friend in the car whom you have not seen for years; you are elated to see her. In this case, the friend in the car is the stressor; your joyful reaction is the stress. Or suppose that the car swerves and seems about to hit you; you experience fear. In this case the oncoming car is the stressor; your fear is the stress.

As you see, a stressor may be negative or positive, happy or sad, uplifting or frightening. It's not even necessary that the stressor take place in the world around you. It may take place only in your mind. If you remember or anticipate an unpleasant happening or a joyful occasion, the thought itself is a stressor, and your reaction to the remembered or anticipated event is the stress.

The stress that results from a happy event is called eustress. As I will discuss later in this book, it is theorized that eustress is physically beneficial. The stress that follows an unhappy event is known simply as stress or distress, and it is this type of stress that evokes the fight-or-flight response, which in turn depresses the immune system.

Fight-or-Flight Response   The body adapts to every mental or emotional reaction automatically—that is, the components of the body change in relation to one another, in order to prepare the body to handle the new conditions. If the new condition is negative, such as fear of injury, the adaptation is the fight-or-flight response, which we share with every other mammal on earth. When a physical danger is perceived, the mind/body takes all the steps necessary—including an increased heart and pulse rate and a flood of adrenaline—so that we can fight to our maximum capability or run away as fast as possible. If the caveman perceived a tiger in the bush, his body automatically got itself ready to fight the animal or run away from it.

Although the fight-or-flight response was intended so that man and other mammals could protect themselves from physical injury, the problem for us is that emotions other than fear of physical injury—such as hurt feelings or any emotional trauma—evoke the identical physical response. And that's true whether we actually experience this fear or trauma or just remember or anticipate it. It also appears that the more dreadfully and intensely the stressor is perceived, the more drastic the body's reaction.

Emotional problems were of no concern in the very early days of human evolution because, in those times, there was no possibility of psychological harm or hurt feelings. And all threats of physical injury were resolved in one way or another in a very short time. Today, the fight-or-flight response is still of vital importance so that we can react quickly to the threat of physical injury, and in short bursts it will do us no harm. However, in this more civilized era, anxiety can last for months, years—even a lifetime—and it is this long-term, unremitting stress that causes the problem. If your business is on the brink of bankruptcy and you are fighting off creditors, or if your spouse has a prolonged serious illness, or if you are constantly striving to satisfy the imagined demands of a parent who has long since died, you can keep yourself in the fight-or-flight condition for a very long time. This may result in severe suppression of the immune system.

Another and more technical way to understand the dangers of prolonged, unremitting stress is to be aware that when the mind/body adapts to what it considers a new and dangerous condition—which, as noted before, can include purely emotional concerns—one of the body's actions in the fight-or-flight response is the release of a flood of hormones into the bloodstream. Some of these hormones may also inhibit or suppress the functions of the immune system. It is theorized that if this weakened condition of the immune system continues for an extended period, any cancer cells that appear during that time and are ordinarily taken out of action by a normal immune system may be able to gain a foothold. The longer the suppressed condition remains, the more time the cancer cells have to join together to form a tumor.

Hans Selye, the preeminent pioneer in stress research, theorized that all of us have only a limited quantity of energy available for our bodies to use to adapt to both physical and mental trauma. If we use too much of it adapting to mental trauma, he said, we may not have enough left to adapt to physical problems, such as illness caused by bacteria, viruses, or foreigners such as cancer cells. All of us, particularly cancer patients, can benefit by reducing mental trauma so that more of our energy will be available to handle our physical needs.

3. What causes cancer?

❧

From the previous chapter, we know that cancer develops when a cancer cell appears *and* the immune system is not sufficiently robust to perform its function. So there are actually two questions related to the cause of cancer: What factors play a part in causing the cancer cell to be produced? And what factors weaken the immune system so that it is unable to destroy that cancer cell?

According to many authorities on this subject, the factors that may affect the production of cancer cells and the strength of the immune system are of three types: (1) hereditary or genetic, (2) environmental, and (3) behavioral.

INHERITED FACTORS

These hereditary or genetic factors are the physical characteristics we have inherited from our parents, from the color of our eyes and hair to the strength or weakness of our immune system. We have no control over this.

It is possible that the immune system we have inherited is so strong that we could live beside the most polluted canal, smoke three packs of cigarettes a day, lead a highly stressful life, and still not develop cancer. On the other hand, our immune system might be so weak that we could develop cancer even under the most ideal physical and mental conditions. Thus, cancer can develop without regard to any factor other than the inherited inadequacy of the immune system or some other genetic error.

ENVIRONMENTAL FACTORS

These factors include the air we breathe, the food we eat, the liquids we drink, the cigarettes we smoke, and all of the other physical circumstances in which we live. Although we can stop smoking, be careful about the food we eat, and try to the best of our ability to be careful about the air we breathe, it's obvious (with the noted exception of tobacco use) that we still have only a limited amount of control over our environment. An environment high in carcinogens (substances that promote cancerous growth) can cause a substantial increase in the number of cancer cells produced.

To illustrate the role played by the environment, assume that John has inherited an immune system of reasonable strength. But suppose he takes up smoking, or gets a job in an asbestos factory (asbestos fibers are known to be carcinogenic), or encounters other environmental conditions that, over the years, cause an unusually large number of cancer cells to appear. It's quite possible that his immune system, strong enough to protect him from a normal number of cancer cells, will not be able to ward off the effects of this more vigorous and persistent attack. Environmental factors caused his body to produce more cancer cells than his immune system could handle, thus tipping a delicate balance.

BEHAVIORAL FACTORS

This category encompasses how we live our lives and how we react to life experiences and events. These factors are known by many names, such as states of mind, attitudes, coping mechanisms, psychological factors, and lifestyles. Although we don't think about it often, we all know that we have a great deal of control over our behavior—our methods of coping. And, as you will see, such control is extremely important to the cancer patient.

As we know, stress depresses the immune system, and the more intense the stress the greater the suppression of the immune system. What we may not have thought about is that our coping style—our behavior—determines the stress we undergo and the amplitude and duration of that stress. It follows then that, if we control our reactions to traumatic events or confine them to a limited period of time, we may be able to avoid the onset of cancer. But more important to the readers of this book, if cancer is already present, our control of the reaction may significantly enhance the possibility of recovery.

Assume that Robert has worked for ten years in an asbestos factory (an environmental factor), where his immune system (an inherited factor) has been sufficiently robust to prevent the development of cancer. However, if Robert's wife leaves him and his children become delinquent, and if he reacts violently to these events over a long time, that reaction to the situation may suppress his immune system so that it is unable to destroy all the cancer cells as they appear.

Notice that it is not the stressors that suppress his immune system; it is his *reaction* to those stressors (his behavior) that does the damage.

Robert has, and we all have, some control over how angry and hurt we will permit ourselves to feel and how long that rage and despair lasts. Robert can take action so that his reaction to the events—the stress he underwent—is less dramatic and won't last so long. Thus his immune system will be less affected and may remain strong enough to ward off the cancer cells as they appear.

The point of this chapter then is to make it very clear:

- That your behavior may have an effect on the course of the illness;
- That you have some control over how you behave;
- That therefore you just may have some control over the course of the illness.

In this book, I will reiterate that lesson in many different ways and also alert you to various situations brought about by cancer which, if they are not recognized, may evoke an automatic unhealthy reaction.

One word of caution. When many cancer patients become aware of the fact that their behavior may have played a part in the onset of the illness, their immediate tendency is to blame themselves for the illness. Also, when they learn that their behavior may be a factor in the fight for recovery, as soon as the illness does not progress as they want it to, they blame themselves for the setback. In chapters 16, 17, and 18 I will explain in detail why neither of these self-blaming reactions makes any sense. You are not to blame for the onset of the illness, and while there are many ways in which you can participate in your fight for recovery, you are not at fault if the illness does not progress as you want it to.

---

4. Is there any way to consciously control my body's internal physical functions?

❦

"There doesn't seem to be any internal process, from the functioning of the organs to the working of a single cell, that a person can't learn to control consciously, provided he has the tools and can cultivate the skills." Those are the words of biofeedback researcher Barbara Brown, and they seem to answer this chapter's question in the affirmative.

This is very good news for the cancer patient; because if it is true, and if we can find the right tools and properly cultivate the skills, perhaps we can strengthen the immune system and direct it to use its full power at the site of the problem to alter the course of the illness toward health. One way to define a Patient Active, then, is a person with cancer who is searching for the right tools and seeking to cultivate the skills to control his or her body's cellular activity—that is, to increase the power of the immune system and alter the course of the disease toward health.

A brief explanation of biofeedback research will help you understand the use of the mind to promote good health. As a starting point, keep in mind that almost all internal functions of our bodies that occur without any effort or thought on our part—such as digestion, blood pressure, heartbeat, and the immune system—are controlled by the involuntary nervous system.

Until biofeedback evolved in the early 1970s, it had been commonly accepted that we had no conscious control over the involuntary nervous system or the seemingly automatic functions it regulated. But biofeedback has demonstrated that we do have some ability to direct these functions.

Most of us believe that the temperature of our skin is one of the many bodily functions that is out of our control—that nothing we can consciously do will raise or lower it. But a biofeedback experiment shows us otherwise. A device that measures skin temperature is placed on some part of the body, such as an arm. The device is attached to a gauge, positioned so the subject can see it.

The subject is then instructed to visualize her arm in a bucket of ice water or some other imaginary freezing situation. As she concentrates on this image, the gauge attached to her arm indicates that her skin temperature is dropping. By just thinking, she has lowered the temperature of her skin—a function she previously believed to be outside of her control. She now realizes she *does* have control of this function if she can find the proper tools and learn how to use them.

The concept illustrated by biofeedback gives rise to one of the most important questions in modern medicine: If we can consciously control our skin temperature and other "automatic" responses, can we control our immune system? No one as yet knows the answer to that question, but we can certainly try. As Dr. Brown said, "We can control any function of the body, if we know how."

Though we in the United States have realized only recently that we have control over the internal workings of our bodies, other cultures have long accepted this. Elmer and Alyce Green of the Menninger Clinic have done considerable research with yogis who can lower their heart rates from sixty to thirty beats per minute in a matter of seconds, and who can reduce blood flow to their limbs through their control of breath and muscle tension. Other researchers who studied Zen meditators in Japan reported finding changes in brain waves resulting from conscious mental effort. The stories in this area are endless. And they all corroborate that we do have control over many, if not all, of the functions controlled by what we have always called the involuntary nervous system.

But don't underestimate or overestimate the power of that statement—or your own power. As yet, no one has worked out a surefire biofeedback or psychological formula that will ensure a cure for cancer or any other disease.

The Patient Active believes the possibility of enhancing the immune system's power makes the effort well worthwhile. But remember, if you work hard for recovery and the illness still doesn't proceed as you want it to, it's not your fault. You did all anyone could do. If you're successful, take all the credit. But if not, it's presumptuous of you to take any of the blame.

---

5. Is cancer always preceded by a traumatic life event six to eighteen months before the diagnosis?

☙

No, not always, but there may be a connection between stressful events and the onset of cancer. A traumatic experience causes stress that depresses the immune system, which in turn may allow cancer to develop. However, as explained in chapter 3, our immune system can be so weak or the carcinogenic conditions around us so severe that cancer can develop even if we live a completely stress-free life. So to say that cancer is *always* preceded by a traumatic event is to fly in the face of the facts.

In the early 1960s, psychiatrists Thomas Holmes and Richard Rahe noticed that an unusually high percentage of cancer patients had experienced relatively severe psychological trauma between six and eighteen months before diagnosis. They hypothesized that if there were a connection between the two events and if they could measure the trauma necessary to weaken the immune system sufficiently to permit the development of illness, they would have a method of predicting who would become ill.

In 1967, they prepared what came to be known as the Holmes-Rahe Social Readjustment Scale—a list of stressful life events, with a numerical value assigned to each corresponding to the severity of its psychological impact. For example, the death of a spouse was assigned the value of 100, while minor violations of the law were rated as 11. Forty other life changes were placed in between, such as troubles with the boss (23), sexual difficulties (40), and marriage (50). Thus, the scale includes both happy and unhappy events.

After preparing the list, Holmes and Rahe conducted a year-long study. They found that among people whose traumatic life events during the preceding year had a cumulative score of 300 or more, 49 percent suffered some type of serious illness soon thereafter. By contrast, only 9 percent of those scoring below 200 became ill during the same period.

The Holmes-Rahe study was followed by a number of similar studies that arrived at many different and often ominous ratios and conclusions. But I believe that the specific numbers and ratios are not important to each of us as individuals except (1) to emphasize and reinforce the belief that stress may play an important part in the onset of illness, and (2) to alert us to be on the lookout for long-term reactions to stressful situations that occurred prior to our diagnosis that may still be depressing our immune systems.

The case of Lynn, an entrepreneur whose partner had forced her out of the business she had started, illustrates these two points. When her business difficulties occurred, Lynn cried and screamed at her partner for as long as he would listen, and then she screamed some more. From then on, that was all she could talk about.

About six months later, Lynn was diagnosed as having cancer, and about six months after that she came to The Wellness Community. But even one year later, after hours of discussion with her participant group (a psychotherapeutic group that meets weekly) about the effect this reaction might be having on her immune system, there was still no way of having a conversation with Lynn that didn't end up with her complaining about her ex-partner. She was obsessed. And that was her immune-depressing condition until the day she died.

Many of Lynn's group-mates felt that she never actually understood the risk she was taking by her inability or un-willingness to give up her hate and need for revenge. If she had acted in a more forgiving way, the outcome of her illness may have been different.

One of the lessons to be learned from Lynn is this: If you have cancer, look back at your life before the diagnosis to see if there was an event or series of events to which you reacted in ways that may have adversely affected your immune system. You can't do anything to change past events, of course, but by examining your past reaction to a traumatic event, you will sense immediately whether you continue to be affected by that event in a way that may still be depressing your immune system.

If you have already let go of the potentially damaging feelings of anxiety, depression, or sorrow—congratulations. But if you are still clinging to them as Lynn did, perhaps it's time for you to take steps to modify those reactions so that they place less pressure on your immune system.

I realize that changing an emotional reaction is not easy, but it can be done. Many cancer patients have learned to do so once they understood that their reactions were jeopardizing their recovery.

What if you have experienced a tragedy such as the sudden loss of a child or spouse? Can you control your reactions to an event so traumatic?

Victors answer this question with another one: How long should we mourn any loss? Of course, everyone will answer that in his or her own way. But Victors constantly remind each other that prolonged grief or any other negative emotion may be having an unwanted effect on their well-being, and that we all have *some* control over how long our emotions last.

Patients Active would suggest that even if you feel like continuing to grieve about an unhappy, unchangeable event in your past, you can "act as if" you have accepted the loss and are no longer upset about it. The "act as if" technique is discussed in detail in chapter 30.

If you just can't stop grieving, try directed visualization (see chapter 32) to intervene between the grief and the resulting negative physical reactions.

---

6. Is there such a thing as a cancer-prone personality?

☙

The words *cancer-prone personality* describe an individual whose habitual negative ways of reacting to life events keep his body in a fight-or-flight condition most of the time, rendering him more vulnerable to cancer.

The first known reference to this personality-based theory appeared nearly 2000 years ago in the writings of the physician Galen. He observed that cheerful women were less prone to cancer than gloomy ones.

Many physicians since Galen's time have observed the relationship between personality traits and the onset of cancer.

Walter H. Walshe, M.D., thoroughly reviewed the literature in his definitive text, *Nature and Treatment of Cancer.* He summarized his findings this way: "Facts of a very convincing character in respect to the agency of the mind and personality in the production of this disease (cancer) are frequently observed. I have myself met cases in which the connection is so clear ... that questioning its reality would have seemed a struggle against reason."

On the other hand, after a thorough review of the literature on the subject, David K. Wellisch, M.D., and Joel Yeager, M.D., of UCLA concluded that "the cancer-prone personality has been elusive and perhaps non-existent." B. H. Fox, M.D., also studied the subject extensively and concluded "that because it is so difficult for science to determine whether there is such a personality, it is doubtful that we will ever know."

Whether such a personality exists or not, suppose you realize that before your diagnosis, you responded to most events in your life in a negative way—and are still doing so. Wouldn't you be wise to try to change?

Ask yourself the following questions:

• Do you invariably and unconsciously react to certain situations in ways that keep you under stress for long periods of time?

• In what types of situations do you usually react negatively?

• Is your negative reaction based on current facts, or on memories of past unpleasant experiences?

• Is there a certain person or persons to whom you react negatively?

• Are you unhappy most of the time?

• Do you believe that you deserve to be unhappy most of the time?

The number of questions is limited only by your imagination. Although the past is your reference point, be sure to couch the questions in terms of the present, because you want to make worthwhile changes *now.*

Your answers may surprise you. Many cancer patients have discovered that their negative reactions were habit and nothing more. With such a revelation, freedom often follows.

If you find that you have been consistently reacting in ways not in your best interest, *don't blame yourself.* Blaming oneself for illness is counterproductive. Chapter 16 will explain why there is no way you can be at fault.

Once you discover a negative personality trait, you will want to change it, and the most efficient way to modify a bad habit is to keep it in your conscious awareness. Habits are reflex actions performed without thought or awareness. But if you are aware that you are about to react to a situation in a way that is not in your best interest, it is likely that—at least some of the time—you will replace that automatic reaction with a more suitable one. Watch yourself and ask your friends and family to help by telling you when they see you acting in a way you want to discontinue.

Don't let anyone convince you that you can't change lifelong habits. It may not be easy, but it can be done.

Stan, a 29-year-old accountant who developed brain cancer, is one illustration of how much people can change. When Stan came to The Wellness Community about three years ago, he could hardly walk or talk. Today, because of the fine medical treatment he received—and, he believes, because of his own efforts to recover—only remnants of these infirmities remain. Over several years, Stan spent a great deal of time talking about his personality and the way he reacted to life, and he made some remarkable discoveries and changes.

Before cancer, Stan says he was not proud of himself or happy with life. His immediate reaction to every situation was to think he was not capable of handling it. He was sure he was a failure.

But in an appearance on a TV show not long ago, Stan showed a much more positive personality.

I've had three brain operations, chemotherapy, and radiation. I've been through a lot in three years. And all I can say is that because of my experiences with cancer and the fact that my family and friends came through for me, I look at myself completely differently today. I was just thinking that I'm actually proud of myself for the first time in many years—way before cancer—and I'm happy with life.

He had changed. He realized that he was the best Stan there was.

It's fair to say that Stan no longer has a cancer-prone personality—if there is such a thing.

Some skilled clinicians believe they have identified certain coping mechanisms that appear in the personalities of a disproportionate number of cancer patients. C. B. Bahnson, Ph.D., found that many cancer patients have a "personality marked by self-containment, inhibition, rigidity, repression, and regression." Lawrence LeShan, Ph.D., observed that many cancer patients are described by friends as being "too good to be true, gentle, fine, thoughtful, and uncomplaining." He wrote, "Cancer patients appear to be compliant, submissive, passive, selfless, and anxious to please in order to avoid being disliked."

As you do some self-evaluating, pay particular attention to your ability to express anger and hostility, and your need to have everybody love you.

Even those of you who are presently healthy might ask yourselves whether you respond to life events in ways that keep you in a cancer-vulnerable fight-or-flight condition. If you are, you might consider making some changes that could be the proverbial stitch in time.

7. Can the many myths that surround cancer inhibit the recovery process?

As you'll see in this and later chapters, although these myths and misconceptions are absurd, they stubbornly persist, often transforming cancer from an illness of the body to a disease of the soul.

To begin, let's define the word *myth*. As we use the term, a myth is a community-held belief that proves to be false once the facts emerge. For example, people believed for a long time that the earth was flat and that if they ventured too far out to sea, they would fall off. All decisions were based upon that "fact." The world was circumscribed with an imaginary boundary, and traffic and cultural exchange between continents were impossible. The world-is-flat myth persisted until Columbus disproved it.

The myths about cancer are as deeply ingrained in our psyches as the myth about the flatness of the earth once was. They come to us from the highest authorities, and they have actually become a part of us. It's vitally important for you to know that if these myths continue to be your basic belief, they can inhibit you from consciously taking actions which may benefit your recovery process, and they may inhibit your mind/body from automatically performing its self-healing functions (see chapter 10 for a discussion of the placebo effect). To say all this another way: *Your acceptance of the myths may make recovery less likely than it might otherwise be.*

At various points in this book, these myths will be discussed in detail:

- Cancer is invincible (chapter 12).
- There is nothing the cancer patient can do to help in the fight for recovery (chapter 13).

- Once the disease is diagnosed, the cancer patient must turn over all control of his life to others (chapter 14).

- Life ends after the diagnosis of cancer (chapter 15).

- The cancer patient is to blame for the illness (chapter 16).

- It is the cancer patient's fault if she is not recovering as quickly as she thinks she should (chapter 17).

At this point, let's concentrate on the myth that cancer is a shameful affliction. At a recent meeting of Wellness Community participants, the question for discussion was: Why is cancer considered shameful and embarrassing? At first, the conversation was as serious as could be. But gradually it became obvious just how ridiculous this particular myth is. As we started to reach for the reasons behind the myth, we all became increasingly silly, and the meeting ended with hearty laughter. From that laughter, we all learned that cancer is no more shameful than any other illness—that cancer is visited on the rich and the poor, the young and the old, the educated and the uneducated, the sanitary and the unsanitary.

All of the participants said they had once been ashamed and embarrassed about having cancer but were no longer. They had lost their shame when they met others who had or had had cancer and who were not ashamed or embarrassed by that fact, and when they learned to discuss cancer openly instead of in whispers.

You are taking the first step toward ridding yourself of any shame you may have about the illness by reading the experiences of the ex-cancer patients in this book. Meeting others with cancer will help, too. Talk about the myths and make fun of them. They deserve it. Try to find some justification for them, as we did in our meeting, and you will see how groundless they are. This way of getting rid of the myths works. I know it does. I've seen it happen over and over again, and it's important.

8. Can the words I use about cancer hinder my fight for recovery?

Many of the words we use about cancer were spawned by misconceptions about the illness. Nearly everywhere, people with cancer are called "cancer victims," and they are said to have a "terminal illness" or a "catastrophic disease." At The Wellness Community, we don't use those terms.

In fact, I didn't want to use the term *cancer patient* in this book, because it suggests passivity and limits the individual's role in life to that of a patient. But I had no real choice. The alternatives were to make up a word like *canceric*— much as a person with diabetes is called a diabetic—or to use the cumbersome phrase *people with cancer.*

The words we use are very important. They fix images and ideas in our minds. The word *victim* describes a person who is helpless in the face of a specific adversity, such as a tornado or a flood. So if we use the words *cancer victim,* we are telling ourselves, with every use of the phrase, that people who have cancer are helpless and doomed.

For the same reason, the term *terminal cancer* is taboo, for it conveys the message that every person with cancer will die of the disease. But not every cancer is terminal, so what benefit is there in characterizing the illness in terms so melodramatic that it takes on the aura of invincibility?

Calling cancer a "catastrophic disease," or the time spent with the illness an "ordeal," is also unnecessary, overly dramatic, and serves no real purpose. You'll find that the phrase "your illness" is never used in this book, either. After all, who would want to own cancer?

Even so, it often takes an effort to get beyond using the negative words that have crept into our language about cancer. Not long ago, a woman named Sharon came into one of our Sharing Groups with a long face and drooping shoulders. She had been operated on five weeks before for colon cancer. Even though she had been told her prognosis was good, in relating her story she described herself as a cancer "victim" and said she had a "catastrophic" and "terminal" disease.

When the Sharing Group leaders suggested that Sharon substitute less melodramatic words, she seemed to resent their observations. However, after she had heard fifteen other personal stories, her demeanor was no longer that of defeat. "I can't believe how wrong I was," Sharon told the group. "My doctor told me I would probably recover and yet I insisted on calling myself a terminal cancer patient, and I probably would have continued to do so if I hadn't met all of you. I don't feel terminal now. What a relief."

So at The Wellness Community, we are very careful about the words we use and the myths that others believe in. We suggest you do the same.

---

9. Is there scientific evidence that emotions can have a beneficial effect on the fight for recovery?

૨

We have known for quite a while, from both anecdotes and scientific evidence, that negative emotions have negative physical results. But while we have had much anecdotal evidence, such as accounts from Norman Cousins, that *positive* emotions can have *positive* effects on our well-being, we are just starting to prove that fact scientifically.

This new thesis is supported by the work of Joan Borysenko, Ph.D., of Harvard University, who found that diabetic patients require less insulin when relaxed than when they are excited. In another study, Christopher Coe, Ph.D., of Stanford University discovered that people who have social support maintain stronger immune systems than those who don't.

At a 1984 conference at Stanford University entitled "How Might the Positive Emotions Affect Physical Health?" James Henry, M.D., of Loma Linda University reported that a shift from feelings of security to feelings of helplessness is accompanied by a rise in certain hormones that depress the power of the immune system, but that *"positive emotions may, in fact, prevent illness by offsetting the damaging consequences of negative emotions"* (emphasis added).

At the same conference, Nicholas Hall, Ph.D., of George Washington Medical School reported on his work with cancer patients who practice positive imagery techniques. "Such patients," he said, "had a rise in the number of disease-fighting lymphocytes in peripheral blood, and also an increase in the level of hormones which augment the immune system."

Research also reveals that even our smiles alter our physical well-being. Paul Ekman, Ph.D., of the University of California, San Francisco, found that when a subject smiled, the immune system was bolstered. He concluded that "states of happiness may reset the [immune system]." William Fry, M.D., of Stanford University, perhaps America's foremost expert on physical reactions provoked by laughter/humor, has demonstrated repeatedly that there is a positive correlation between healthy hormonal activity and laughter/humor. He has conducted blood tests showing that the immune system is strengthened in subjects after a session of laughter.

Research into multiple-personality disorder also has added credence to the theory that personality affects health. Bennett G. Braun, M.D., has described several of these cases in the *American Journal of Clinical Hypnosis.* The first multiple-personality subject had one personality who was color-blind and another who was not. In the second case, a woman had more than five personalities, all of whom had diabetes, "which required variable amounts of insulin depending on which personality had control of the body and the emotional stresses." Thus, the personality determined how her body responded to the illness.

For our purposes, the remarkable aspect of this mental condition is that one of the personalities can have a set of physical reactions, attributes, or disabilities substantially different from those of the other personalities, though they're all in the same body. What better evidence of the effect of mental state on physical well-being?

The field of hypnosis provides further scientific evidence of the mind's ability to control the body. With hypnosis—which is actually just another way of utilizing our mental ability to control bodily functions—warts can be removed, allergies cured, migraines relieved, bleeding controlled in hemophiliacs, and many other bodily processes altered, impeded, and induced. More important to cancer patients, Howard Hall, Ph.D., of Pennsylvania State University has reported on clinical tests demonstrating that changes in mental activity induced by hypnosis have actually altered and enhanced the effectiveness of the immune system.

So now we know from both anecdotes and science that quality of life is an important facet of total well-being and well worth striving for as part of the fight for recovery.

---

10. What is the placebo effect, and how can I use it in my fight for recovery?

ॐ

If a physician believes you will feel better if you receive some type of medicine or treatment—even though he doesn't believe you actually need it—he will sometimes prescribe an inert substance, such as a sugar pill. That harmless "medication"—a placebo—somehow relieves the symptoms. The same substance, taken without a belief in its curative powers, would have no effect at all. Your recovery, based on nothing more than your trust in the physician and the belief that the medicine will cure you, is called the placebo effect.

One case history, reported by Bruno Klopfer, Ph.D., is recited in many writings about the placebo effect because it illustrates so well the power of the phenomenon. In the 1950s, the drug Krebiozen was being tested as a cure for cancer. Dr. Klopfer had it administered to one of his patients with advanced cancer. The patient, who was approaching death before the administration of the drug, made a remarkable recovery and returned to many of his normal activities. Soon thereafter, testing proved the drug to be completely without curative power, and when the patient became aware of that fact, he again became "terminally ill."

At that point (and in a time when lawsuits were less threatening than they are today), Dr. Klopfer decided to take a chance. He told the patient he had obtained a new and better formula of Krebiozen and believed this drug might effect a cure. He then injected the patient with large amounts of sterile water, a placebo. Once again, the patient made an unbelievable recovery and resumed many of his normal pursuits. But soon thereafter, the patient learned of the ruse and died.

The point here is that the patient's belief in something (although it wasn't true) stimulated his body to take the actions necessary to correct the malady. If the patient had not believed in the placebo's power, his body would not have taken these curative actions. When he lost faith in the medicine, his body stopped doing those things that protected him from the illness.

There are literally hundreds of studies showing that the administration of a placebo often works to cure the patient. As psychologists J. Critelli and K. Neuman have written, "The placebo was once the mainstay of medical practice. Few remedies used by physicians had any specific effect on the disorders for which they were prescribed, yet patients nonetheless improved due to the placebo effect... which stimulated the patient's innate capacity for self-repair."

Herbert Benson, M.D., of Harvard University called attention to this in the *Harvard Medical School Letter*: "In the past various useless agents were believed to be effective against disease: lizard's blood, crushed spiders, putrid meat, crocodile dung, bear fat, fox lungs, eunuch fat, and moss scraped from the skull of a hanged criminal. Likewise, cupping, blistering, plastering, and leeching had their day. When *both* physician and patient believed in them, these remedies could indeed have been helpful some of the time."

Throughout medical history, the placebo effect has been said to apply when the patient believed something that wasn't true. But now, the vitally important question is, can you get your body to take the actions necessary for recovery (the placebo effect) without tricking it? In his book *Anatomy of an Illness*, Norman Cousins answers the question affirmatively as follows:

> An understanding of the way the placebo works may be one of the most significant developments in medicine in the 20th century. It is doubtful whether the placebo—or any drug for that matter —would get very far without a patient's robust will to live.... The placebo has a role to play in transforming the will to live from a hypothetical conception to a physical reality and governing force.... *What we see ultimately is that the placebo isn't really necessary and the mind can carry out its difficult and wonderous mission unprompted by little pills.... The placebo is the emissary between the will to live and the body. But the emissary is expendable.* If we can liberate ourselves from tangibles, we can connect hope and the will to live directly to the ability of the body to meet great

threats and challenges. The mind can carry out its ultimate functions and powers over the body without the illusion of material intervention. [Emphasis added.]

The credo of the Patient Active in regard to this issue is: "I know that my total being, including my brain and my body, is powerful enough and has sufficient resources so that under all but the most unfortunate circumstances, it can and does automatically return me to health. I also know that it can be tricked by a placebo into using that power to effect a recovery. I will now do everything in my power without deceiving myself to consciously release the power of recovery that I know is inherent in my body/mind so that I may recover from cancer."

How do you release that power? As yet, there is no definitive answer. But Patients Active are aware that the combination of hope, the will to live, the willingness to accept life as it is, and to enjoy it to the greatest extent possible are a wonderful place to start. Making the effort, being a part of the fight for recovery—just trying—may be all that's necessary.

I know of no better description of the potential efficacy of the placebo effect than a statement made jointly by Norman Cousins and Barrie R. Cassileth, M.D., of the University of Pennsylvania, printed on a *Los Angeles Times* editorial page in October 1985. Their joint article grew out of a report of a study conducted by Dr. Cassileth published in the *New England Journal of Medicine* earlier in that year. Dr. Cassileth had studied 359 patients with advanced cancer. These patients had answered questions concerning psychological, social, and emotional matters that had been "found, in previous investigations, to predict longevity or survival."

The study, based on one interview with each advanced cancer patient within two to eight weeks of the diagnosis of the illness, concluded that "analysis does not support the existence of relation between the psychosocial factors studied and survival or time to recurrence of the disease." In other words, the study found that neither the psychological state nor the activities of the patient had any effect on the biological course of the illness.

In an editorial in the same issue of the medical journal, Marcia Angell, M.D., concluded that previous studies suggesting an actual connection between mind and body were so flawed as to be unreliable, and that to believe that the mind had any effect on physical well-being was "folklore."

Dr. Cassileth's study received much media attention and caused much consternation and despair among cancer patients. The joint statement by Cousins and Cassileth attempted to counter such misunderstanding. They wrote:

> The current public controversy over the relationship between emotions and health has placed the authors of this article on opposite sides. Much of the controversy, however, has its origin in serious misunderstandings of our basic positions. What concerns us especially is that these misunderstandings can produce public confusion and may cause harm to patients who are trying to mobilize their resources in the fight against disease.
>
> The confusion grew out of press reports concerning the article "Psychosocial Correlates of Survival in Advanced Malignant Disease," written by Barrie R. Cassileth and colleagues and published in the *New England Journal of Medicine.* Some of the reports and comments incorrectly interpreted the study's results to mean that positive attitudes have no value in a strategy for effective treatment of illness.
>
> Cassileth's study, however, was not concerned with disease in general but with advanced cancer in particular. Cassileth wrote: "Our study with advanced, high-risk malignant diseases suggests that the inherent biology of the disease alone determines the prognosis, overriding the potentially mitigating influence of psychosocial factors.

This means that in advanced cancer, biology overwhelms psychology. It does not mean the emotions and health are unrelated. It does not mean that emotions and attitudes play no role in the treatment or well-being of ill people.

In any case, high-risk cancer accounts for a very small percentage of all illness in the United States. The fact that positive attitudes or emotions cannot be expected to reverse or cure untreatable cancer does not mean they have no value in the large majority of illnesses. *Indeed, positive attitudes may play a significant role in optimizing medical treatment. Even in advanced malignancies, positive attitudes of patients not only can enhance the environment of treatment, but can have a beneficial effect on the quality of life of patients. Physicians have always believed that a strong will to live helps a patient's chances of combatting serious disease.* [Emphasis added.]

In an analogous fashion, Norman Cousins' work has been grossly simplified. His *Anatomy of an Illness,* first published in the *New England Journal of Medicine,* and his public statements concerning the complex relationship between mental attitude and physical health, have been reduced in some quarters to the absurd notion that laughter can cure cancer.

Cousins used laughter as a metaphor for the full range of the positive emotions, including hope, love, faith, a strong will to live, determination and purpose. He also stressed the importance of the patient-physician partnership in effective medical care.

We hope the following points will dispel the confusion, as well as clarify our points of view. Rather than being diametrically opposed, we share a common understanding and perspective.

Emotions and health are closely related. It has

been known for many years that negative emotions and experiences can have a deleterious effect on health and can complicate medical treatment. Not as well-known is the connection between positive attitudes and the possible enhancement of the body's healing system. This relationship is now the subject of study at a number of medical research centers.

It is likely that numerous emotional and physical factors, many of them yet to be delineated, influence health and disease, probably in different ways for different individuals. There is no single, simple factor that causes or cures cancer and other major illnesses.

Even where positive attitudes and a good mental outlook cannot influence the physical outcome, they can and do affect the quality of life. Few things are more important in the care of seriously ill patients than their mental state and the general environment in which they have to be treated. Unfortunately, human beings are not able to exercise control over all of their biological and disease processes. Therefore, they should not be encouraged to believe that positive attitudes are a substitute for competent medical attention.

The reciprocal mind/body relationship is complex. We must be aware equally of both the potential power and the limitations of attitudes in their effects on health and disease.

To sum up, then, research now being done in many fields lends credence to the thesis that psychological attitudes, states of mind, social conditions, and emotional reactions may play a part in aiding or inhibiting the recovery from illness. Therefore Patients Active do everything in their power to increase the mind's involvement in the recovery process and they do it even though they may be skeptical about the results of their efforts, because they *hope* that their efforts will be beneficial. And without hope, there is nothing.

So try it. Even if it doesn't work exactly the way you want it to, at least you are taking back some control in your life. And as we shall soon see, that's invaluable to the recovery process.

---

11. Can expectations as to the outcome of the illness have an effect on recovery?

❧

No one can answer that question with any degree of certainty. However, much has been written about the thesis known as self-fulfilling prophecy, which augurs well for the patient who *expects* to recover.

This thesis suggests that if we believe in the inevitability of a certain result, we will act either consciously or unconsciously to ensure the expected result. We have all heard stories of the voodoo witch doctor who prophesizes that a particular tribal member will die at a given time, and turns out to be right. It's quite likely that the unfortunate victim so believed in the inevitability of the prophecy that he unconsciously instructed his body to die at the appointed hour. In essence, this is the placebo effect in reverse and a perfect example of the self-fulfilling prophecy.

Various researchers have applied this thesis to cancer patients, theorizing that people who expect to recover are more likely to do so than individuals who believe the illness is fatal. I have observed that cancer patients with high expectations of recovery appear to live much happier lives while fighting the illness than those who expect to die, and this in itself may have a beneficial effect on the recovery process. And many ex-cancer patients indicate that there never was a doubt in their mind they would recover.

Robert K. Merton, Ph.D., an authority on the subject, has written that "the self-fulfilling prophecy is, in the beginning, a *false* definition of a situation, evoking a new behavior which makes the originally false definition come *true.*" If a cancer patient expects the illness to be fatal, which may be a false premise, perhaps she unconsciously directs her body to stop fighting the illness; this new behavior results in the outcome originally prophesied. This may work in reverse for the patient who expects to recover.

The cancer patient may benefit, then, from having *as many positive expectations and as few negative expectations as possible.* Of course, you cannot change an expectation that is a part of your belief system by the stroke of an intention; but many cancer patients have changed from believing that their illness was sure to be fatal, to believing and hoping that recovery is a real possibility. They have achieved this with the help of their friends and other cancer patients, and by using the "act as if" technique (see chapter 30).

Ryan, 45, who has been recovered from colon cancer for over twelve years, is one example. He says:

> When I was told I had colon cancer, my doctors told me to get my affairs in order since my time was quite limited. And I believed them. With all my heart and soul, I believed them.
>
> But one morning I woke up feeling better than I had in a long time, and I decided, then and there, that I wasn't going to give up without a fight. Even though I believed I was going to die, because they told me so, I decided that recovery was a possibility and that I was going to do everything I could to make that happen. And although I had always been a very private person, I went right downstairs and

announced this to my wife and children. I also told all my friends that I *knew* that the treatments I was receiving were going to cure me.

I kept saying this over and over again, even when I felt as sick as a dog. After a while, every time I talked about my recovery—and I would talk about it a lot—I would feel a thrill of hope run through me. I also started to talk about my plans for the future, even though there was a part of me that "knew" I was kidding myself. And the more I talked about the future, the more possible it seemed that there would be a future for me. I don't know if that had anything to do with my recovery, but it sure made me feel better.

If you have cancer, why don't you stop reading now and think about the ways you would act, the plans you would make, and the things you would say if you expected to recover. Then go out and say them and do them. That's "acting as if," and it may just fool your autonomic nervous system into working as hard as it can for your recovery. This does not preclude discussing your fear that the results won't be as you hope—but don't dwell on your doubts.

Don't be discouraged if results take a while. However, if you've given this approach a full try and it doesn't work for you, don't blame yourself. It doesn't work for everybody. Try something else.

Expectations can also be important in dealing with the treatment for cancer. If you *expect* chemotherapy to cause nausea and vomiting, it probably will. Many cancer patients become ill on the way to the doctor's office at the mere *thought* of the treatment. (It's interesting to note that although cancer is the enemy and chemotherapy is a friend, they are painted with the same hateful brush.) But just as the body reacts negatively to a negative thought, perhaps it will react positively to the thought that you will have no nausea from the treatment. Try to view the treatment as an aid to recovery, not an enemy. (You also might want to meditate, using visualization techniques, before, during, and after chemotherapy or radiation; a script for chemotherapy or radiation meditation appears in chapter 34.)

After the treatment, "act as if" and "talk as if" the chemo didn't make you very uncomfortable. Your subconscious has a great deal of difficulty remembering what the nausea felt like, but it has no difficulty remembering in detail every word you said about how you felt. If you describe your discomfort in less dramatic terms, perhaps your memory will be shaped to meet the relatively mild description.

This may not be an easy or even a natural course of action. It's difficult not to complain when you really have something to complain about. In times of discomfort, we all want to describe the problem in terms that evoke sympathetic responses from others, and we deserve all the help we can get when we don't feel well.

But take the case of Geoff, who decided to "act as if" the chemicals he was ingesting were "friends and an elixir with magical properties," in the hope that doing so would minimize the side effects of the treatment and maximize his body's reaction to it. This change in his attitude did not evolve unconsciously; it was a decision carefully arrived at, after he had been advised that such a step might be helpful. He considered the advice, saw he had nothing to lose, and decided to accept it.

Geoff then started to think and speak of his treatments not as horrendous, dreadful times of torture with awful sickness and nausea as the inevitable result; instead, he spoke as if they were a method of fighting for recovery that had only irritating, not sickening, side effects. And gradually, his perception of the treatment changed. The unpleasant effects diminished. This won't happen to everyone, but it's worth a try.

Tim is another example of expectations coming to fruition. He fought lymphoma for several years and has been symptom-free since December 1982. He always considered chemotherapy his friend and ally, picturing it as a vat of liquid that would disintegrate unhealthy cells to make room for healthy ones. And it never made him sick. He always expected to recover, and told everybody just that.

For Tim, things seem to be working out fine today, and perhaps his expectations had something to do with it. Perhaps his prophecy of recovery was self-fulfilling. And perhaps—just perhaps—you can experience the same results.

II
DEALING WITH REACTIONS
TO CANCER

❧

12. Sometimes I find it hard to believe that there is always room for hope.

॰

There is much reason to have hope, although the mythology of cancer has fooled almost everyone into believing otherwise. As a matter of fact, it's unreasonable and unrealistic *not* to have hope.

Knowledge of cancer recovery statistics is the first springboard from which hope is launched. Data published by the American Cancer Society in its 1985/1986 bulletin, *Cancer Facts and Figures*, indicate that 40 to 50 percent of all people who have cancer recover from the illness. There are 5 million Americans alive today who have a history of cancer, and the diagnosis of 3 million of them was made more than five years ago. Most of these 3 million are considered completely recovered, meaning that they have no evidence of the illness and have the same life expectancy as a person who has never had cancer. That's right: *they have the same life expectancy as if they had never had cancer.* All of our participants are well aware that statistics can be interpreted in a great many ways, and they have chosen to interpret them in the same way that the American Cancer Society does—as an indication of progress and hope for the future.

In August 1985 in the *Los Angeles Times,* Eddie Reed, M.D., special assistant to the director of the National Cancer Institute (Division of Cancer Treatment), discussed the statistics of cancer patient survival as follows: "Thirty years ago, advanced cancer was uniformly fatal. Today, impressive cure rates are seen in an increasing number of cancers (testicular cancer, 90 percent; and Hodgkin's disease, 80 percent). These improvements are due to advances in cancer chemotherapy and radiotherapy." Dr. Reed confirmed that at least 40 to 50 percent of patients diagnosed as having cancer in 1985 will completely recover from the illness with the help of chemo-therapy, radiation, and surgery.

So if 3 million people in the United States have already triumphed over cancer, and if 40 to 50 percent of all people who develop cancer in any given year will eventually van-quish the illness, there is certainly every reason for every cancer patient—including you—to have hope. *There is no type of cancer that does not have some recovery rate, and therefore hope for recovery is realistic and reasonable.*

The Patient Active knows that hope improves the quality of life—that cancer patients who have hope for recovery are happier than those who are resigned to a short, unpleasant future. And they recognize that an improved quality of life can have a beneficial effect on the recovery process. Few researchers have better summarized the effect hope can have on recovery than Fred O. Henker, M.D., a professor of psychia-try at the University of Arkansas. At a 1984 meeting of the American Psychiatric Association, after describing various as-pects of the process of recovery from illness, Henker con-cluded with this pithy statement: "Whether we acknowledge the influence of hope or not, it's real, and it may even deter-mine the life or death outcome of the patient." I have yet to meet a physician who does not agree with that statement.

The importance of hope has become such an accepted part of total cancer patient care that Louis A. Gottschalk, M.D., professor of psychiatry and human behavior at the University of California, Irvine, has developed tests to determine the individual's amount of hope. These hope scales were used in one study of twenty-seven patients whose cancer had spread and who were receiving X-ray treatment. The results indi-cated that those with a greater amount of hope lived longer than those without hope.

The key question here is, how can the cancer patient achieve hope? You can foster hope by meeting or becoming aware of ex-cancer patients—the more the merrier (see chapter 37); by keeping up your social contacts (see chapter 24); by paying attention to recovery statistics; by deriding myths and fables that surround cancer and recognizing that they don't apply to you; by becoming aware, at your most conscious level, that as long as statistics show that even one person recovers from the type of cancer you have, there is every reason to hope you will be that one; and, finally, by "acting as if" you have hope (see chapter 30).

So take all of these actions. Go out of your way to be with other cancer patients and fight to keep up as many social contacts as you had before the diagnosis. And talk and act as if you have hope, even if you don't. The results can be impressive. I have seen it happen many times. It may happen for you.

There is no way to examine hope in a cancer patient's life without recognizing the possibility of false hope. When I decided to start The Wellness Community, some people argued that such a program would foster false hope. Frankly, at first, I gave these thoughts serious consideration, but then I realized that these critics erroneously believed that our program would tell cancer patients we "guaranteed" they would get well if they followed our advice. Nothing could be further from the truth. We have always known there is no such thing as a sure cure. Promises that "if you do what we tell you, you *will* get well" are not messages of false hope; they're either fraud or stupidity.

Even Norman Cousins was concerned about creating false hope when he wrote *Anatomy of an Illness* about his fight against a life-threatening illness. He said, "I have not written in any detailed way about my illness...largely because I was fearful of creating false hopes in other persons similarly afflicted."

Cousins was worried that people who had the same disease would believe that if they indulged in large doses of laughter and vitamin C as he did, they would be *guaranteed* of getting well. He took great pains in his book not to create the illusion that there are any promises of recovery, while emphasizing that there is always room for hope.

Actually, there is no such thing as false hope. All cliches have some truth in them, and the pertinent cliche here is, "Where there's life, there's hope."

Bernard Siegel, M.D., a Yale physician who has written

extensively about the psychological and social aspects of cancer treatment, was once asked by a cancer patient, "Can I get
well?" He responded, "Of course you can. Statistics may be
against you, but there's no reason you can't get well." Dr.
Siegel later recalled,

> There's no false hope in a patient's mind.... If one
> person ever got well with a certain disease, then I
> have the right to suggest that another one could. I
> also have the right to suggest that the patient could
> be the first.... I teach patients to be survivors.

Up to this point, we have discussed hope only in terms of
complete recovery. But even for patients who have accepted
the inevitability of something other than recovery, there can
be hope for joy, love, and involvement in life. Just as life does
not end with the diagnosis of cancer, life does not end when
the possibility of recovery becomes remote. Life goes on as
long as life goes on.

Finally, although no one can promise complete recovery,
hope is there for the taking. And with hope comes an improved quality of life, which is a reasonable goal in itself.

---

13. Am I helpless in my fight for recovery?

❧

You are not helpless. There are many actions you as a cancer
patient can take to fight for your own recovery. As a matter of
fact, you are the most important member of the team fighting
for your recovery.

However, with very few exceptions, every cancer patient

experiences feelings of extreme helplessness in the face of cancer at one time or another. In fact, many people—including some physicians—erroneously believe that when cancer is the diagnosis, patients have no alternative but to place themselves in the hands of the health professionals and passively wait and hope that they will be successful in curing them.

Too often, people react to the onset of cancer like a mechanically unskilled driver whose car breaks down. The driver has no alternative but to call a mechanic and then stand by, watch, and hope that the mechanic knows what he's doing. Many cancer patients deal with their bodies the same way—by consulting someone who can "fix" bodies, usually called "Doctor," and doing nothing but watching and hoping that the doctor will succeed.

But the human body/mind is not like an automobile, which, if damaged or malfunctioning, remains that way until it is fixed. Our bodies are exquisite, complex organisms that (except in the most extreme situations) perform everything necessary to maintain or return themselves to their normal state without help from any outside source.

When we develop one of the more than one hundred diseases known as cancer, our immune system does its best to rid the body of the illness. The Patient Active does everything in his or her power to beef up these efforts in the hope or belief that the more powerful the immune system, the more likely the chances of success.

That's why Patients Active use the word *recover* instead of *cure.* From the patient's point of view, *cure* is a passive word ("I hope somebody will 'fix' me or 'cure' me), while *recover* is an active word ("I will do everything I can to 'recover,' with the help of my physician"). Also, they always call themselves *participants,* never *victims.* Victims watch. Participants participate.

Until recently, however, the perception that the cancer patient was helpless was largely accurate. Yet now, because of considerable research into the effect that emotions, attitudes, and other coping mechanisms have on the body, we know that the patient can play an important role in the fight for recovery so that two experts—the physician and the patient—are engaged in the battle instead of only one. Sad to say, this fact is not widely known.

If you have cancer, you are taking action in regard to recovery whether you know it or not. You are either fighting actively to recover or you are waiting for someone else to cure you. Think about it. Are you being active or passive about your recovery?

More and more individuals who consider themselves recovered from cancer believe that their active participation played an important part in their recovery. One such Patient Active is Phil, a 57-year-old real estate developer who had spent the days immediately after receiving the diagnosis talking about suicide. He had late-stage lymphoma, cancer of the lymphatic system, and his doctor had told him his chances of recovery were slim.

Phil, like many other people with cancer, found life after the diagnosis unbearable. Weak and discouraged, he often would burst into tears. He had given up, sure he was going to die soon. Although he had a loving family and friends, he felt alone. He wouldn't let them be with him. They couldn't understand—*they* didn't have cancer; *they* weren't doomed to die.

But Phil's wife, a registered nurse, wanted the old Phil back and was willing to try anything. After much effort, she prevailed on him to try The Wellness Community program. Although he was depressed and could hardly walk, and was still sure he was going to die, Phil began to fight for recovery. He joined a participant group, did directed visualization, changed his diet, began to learn about cancer, took back control of many areas of his life, made sure he was with a lot of cancer patients, and permitted his family to once again treat him as a friend.

As time went on, a remarkable transformation took place. Phil's despair gave way to hope. The crying spells vanished and he started to enjoy life for the first time in many months. His physical condition started to improve.

Today, several years later, Phil is happy, energetic, involved—and without symptoms. He is back at work full-time except when he thinks he is working more than is good for him. Since his cancer, he is more protective of his health than ever before. He wants to do everything he can to make sure that he lives as long as possible and that he enjoys each day to the fullest.

Phil is convinced that his participation in his fight for recovery played an invaluable role in his recovery. "I don't believe I would have survived if I had not had wonderful medical treatment, and if I had not taken the actions I did to help myself get well. Without either I was a goner."

Phil learned some very important lessons and made some very important choices. *Choosing to be a Patient Active is actually not a single monumental choice; it is a series of small decisions to fight for recovery, rather than letting nature take its course.*

Because Phil's early negative thoughts may reflect some of your own feelings at this time, it's important for you to know that most cancer patients, when they first hear the diagnosis, are like Phil, and perhaps like you—despondent, frightened, sure they have no chance of recovery, and certain they are helpless. But all that changes when they learn the facts, give up the myths, and begin to act as Patients Active. Yes, they are concerned and anxious, and many times frightened and apprehensive. But they are fighting, and not fighting alone. They know they have a chance and are not helpless. They act optimistic and, to the best of their ability, energetic and because of all that, life becomes more livable, more pleasant. The juices start to flow. And all of that is available to you. I know it is. I have seen it happen to hundreds of cancer patients just like you.

14. Cancer seems to have stripped me of all control of my life.

❧

Most people with cancer know only too well the feelings of helplessness brought on by the loss of control caused by their illness. A cancer-imposed dependence on others after a lifetime of independence and self-sufficiency often provokes such feelings. Routine tasks become monumental undertakings. Those who depended on you in the past have now become those on whom you depend. Almost everything is different. And no matter what you do, all this will continue to some extent until you recover.

Many cancer patients who have lost some control over their lives—in many cases temporarily—believe that they have lost *all* control *forever.* They further believe that depression and despair are the only normal reactions to the loss of any control, and that there is nothing they can do to retain or regain control of any part of their lives.

But many cancer patients just like you have traded helplessness for involvement and despair for hope, when they understand:

1. That they have retained more control than they thought they had.

2. That there are many ways a Patient Active can regain much of the control he or she has given up.

3. That every cancer patient can learn to accept, with some degree of equanimity, the loss of control he or she can't retain.

The cancer patient's loss of control and the resulting feelings of helplessness have been well described by Neil Fiore, Ph.D., a practicing clinical psychologist. In 1974, Fiore was diagnosed as having cancer that had metastasized to his lungs. He fought the illness with a fine medical team and his own active participation. After surgery and a stringent treatment of chemotherapy, he is without symptoms of any kind. In the *New England Journal of Medicine,* he wrote:

> Anyone with serious illness will experience some sense of depression and helplessness. For patients with cancer, however, the sense of helplessness is magnified both by the universal belief that cancer is equivalent to death, to being a victim and to suffering, and by the vast technical expertise that has been brought to bear on combatting the disease, which tends to take all decisions about treatment out of the patient's hands.... Cancer patients do not feel effective or even have control over their own bodies. Their very cells seem to be rebelling and going crazy.

In an article titled "Group Psychotherapy with Cancer Patients," M. Lynn Rickert, Ph.D., and Andrew Koffman, Ph.D., make the following comment:

> Virtually all cancer patients perceive a painful loss of control over their lives. In contrast to many other diseases, the nature of cancer is such that patients generally believe they are unable to affect its course. They believe that nothing they can do, or refrain from doing, will alter the outcome of the illness.

This loss of control and resulting feeling of helplessness are serious problems to the cancer patient. They lead to a giving-up behavior and loss of the will to live, two potent negative stressors that may prevent purposeful activity to recover and hinder automatic internal curative processes.

At this point, it's important to know that all negative

stress is the result of remembering, experiencing, or antic-
ipating a situation that we believe can harm us either mentally or physically, and *over which we have no control.* If we
believe we are in control of a situation—that is, if we can
prevent it from harming us physically or mentally—anxiety
vanishes. Thus, if I can control the discussion with the boss
so he won't fire me, or the confrontation with a robber so he
won't hurt me, or the opinions of my friends so they will
always respect and admire me, I will have no stress.

This concept is important because it justifies working so
hard to retain control, although there are times when you
must accept some loss of control. And just making the decision to continue fighting to retain control—or to concede
that there is an area of control that is reasonable to give up—
relieves a great deal of anxiety.

Of course, if the "deal" you have made with God or the
universe is that life is good only on your terms, and your
terms are that you will always be in full control, then you will
find any loss of control unacceptable. If, on the other hand,
you are aware that the amount of control you have, like everything else in life, ebbs and flows, then you can accept the loss
of some control with a certain amount of equanimity. The
ultimate control—how you perceive the event—is yours.
That's a far healthier state of affairs.

The concept that loss of control can impede the fight for
recovery is also based on many human and animal studies. In
one of these human studies, Steven Locke, M.D., divided a
group of healthy males into three groups: (1) those with few
life stressors; (2) those with many life stressors who responded with high anxiety (had little control); and (3) those
with many life stressors who responded with low anxiety
(had much control).

Not surprisingly, Dr. Locke found that the "many
stressors/much control" group had stronger immune systems
than the "many stressors/little control" group. What surprised
everyone is that they also had stronger immune systems than

even the "few stressors" group. Obviously then, its not the stressors that cause the problem; it's the way we react to the stressors—the lack of control—that does the dirty work.

In another human study Arthur Schmale, Ph.D., and Howard Iker, M.D., surveyed fifty-one women who had just taken a test to determine if they had cervical cancer before the results of the tests were known. Their study revealed that 61 percent of the women who felt they had little control over their lives had cancer, while only 24 percent of the women who felt in control of their lives had cancer—more evidence to buttress the belief that the loss of control may play a part in the onset of cancer and therefore can quite possibly have an effect on the recovery process.

Animal studies have been even more conclusive. L. S. Sklarr, Ph.D., and H. Anisman, Ph.D., injected three groups of mice with cancer cells. One group was then exposed to electric shocks from which they could escape by jumping over a barrier; they had complete control over the stressor. The mice in the second group were exposed to random shocks over which they had no control. The third group was never shocked. The researchers then watched the growth of the tumors, and found that the tumor growth in the mice receiving *uncontrollable* shocks was significantly greater than that of the other two groups. On the other hand, they found no significant differences in tumor growth between the group that received no shocks and the group that received controllable shocks.

The researchers concluded that *controllable stress is the same as no stress at all,* at least as far as the immune system is concerned. They also concluded that since the mice that experienced uncontrolled stress had tumor growth significantly greater than either of the two other groups, it was the uncontrollable stress that depressed the immune system, leaving the mice more exposed to the growth of cancer cells. Thus, *uncontrolled stress may be a significant factor in the development of, and possibly the recovery from, cancer.*

What can you do to retain and maintain the control you have, and to regain as much as possible of the control you have given up?

The first step is to make a list of the areas of control you have given up. In other words, what decisions are now made for you that you had always made for yourself? Simply preparing this list will make you aware of the awesome amount of control you had before the diagnosis and how much you still have.

Treat this list very seriously. Be specific about what you have given up. You will probably be surprised to find you have relinquished control in areas where you needn't have. This first list, of course, suggests a second: What have you given up that you can take back?

Then it's time to begin taking control one step at a time, starting with the easy ones. To begin with, you can immediately take control of one significant part of your life—deciding exactly what you will and won't eat.

NUTRITION

Many authorities believe that nutrition is one of the most important parts of the fight for recovery. The United States Department of Health and Human Services, for example, has published a book entitled *Eating Hints, Recipes and Tips for Better Nutrition During Cancer Treatment.* You have everything to gain and nothing to lose by taking an active part in deciding what you will and won't eat. You will not only feel less helpless, you will probably improve your physical condition as well.

In order to control your nutrition intelligently, you should learn as much about proper eating as you can. There must be at least a thousand books about that subject, and perhaps 10 percent of them are slanted toward cancer patients. Educating yourself is the first important step in taking control. And then every time you eat a healthy food because it's good for you, or say "no thank you" to taboo food, you are taking control.

EXERCISE

Another area that is comparatively easy to handle is exercise. Find out if it will help you recover. Get information from your physician, from the American Cancer Society, or from books on the subject. In an article in the journal *Advances* (Fall 1984), Wesley E. Sime, director of the Stress Psychology Laboratory at the University of Nebraska, reviewed the literature and reported that exercise has much the same effect on the immune system as meditation does. If you believe exercise will help, start becoming physically active. If it seems pointless to you, don't do it. Make up your own mind. That's making a choice, taking control.

KNOWLEDGE OF THE ILLNESS

Next, what do you know about the illness diagnosed in your case? Can you discuss it with your doctor knowledgeably? If not, maybe you should do something about that. This is not to say that you should tell your doctor what to do, but shouldn't you be in on the decision-making process? (chapter 48 will look further at your relationship with your doctor.)

Many studies indicate that it can be beneficial for the cancer patient to be knowledgeable about the illness. A study by Anita Stewart, Ph.D., of the Rand Corporation came to that conclusion. In "Measuring the Ability to Cope with Serious Illness," she reported:

> Some [researchers] suggest that patients who have information about the amount of discomfort to be expected from a noxious procedure are able to tolerate the discomfort more easily. Another researcher found that having information about the physical sensations to expect during a stressful medical procedure can reduce the distress. Another found that providing patients with information about what symptoms to expect reduced complica-

tions following a heart attack. Surgical patients who
were told about postoperative pain and what could
be done about it required only one half as much
postoperative narcotics.

Dr. Stewart also reported that studies that have found
that allowing patients to make choices about daily matters
(such as which arm to take blood from), combined with
information about the procedure, resulted in better health, a
heightened sense of well-being, and longer survival, as well as
less stress and anxiety.

As well as *retaining* control, you might also consider
regaining some of the control that you've lost. To find areas of
control you want to regain, go back to the lists you made. You
will probably find many more areas where you can regain
control than you expect. But don't be unreasonable. If you
take on more than you can handle, you can impede the recovery process and make life unbearable for those around you.

What are you to do now? Up to this point, you have been
counseled to take back control, to make choices, to choose
between alternatives—all of which are aggressive, affirmative suggestions. But now you've been urged to use caution
and reasonableness as well, which illustrates that the course
of action you take as a Patient Active is a fine line—aggres-
sively taking back control while not biting off more than you
can chew.

Combining these two seemingly contradictory guidelines
results in the following recommendation: *Do everything in
your power to accentuate all conduct that you believe may
be conducive to your recovery, and eliminate all habits that
may be interfering with that process.*

This advice—obvious yet seemingly difficult to live up
to—takes on its proper importance when you realize that in
order to follow it, you must examine alternatives to reactions
that have always been automatic. Such examination alone—
just assessing the prospective behavior to see if it is bad or
good for you—can result in your having more control of your

life than ever before. It will move the decision-making process from the unconscious to the conscious, from the instinctive to the purposeful, from the reflexive to the deliberate.

You will decide how you want to react to a specific life event, based on current facts rather than upon memories of past experiences. You will decide whether the responses you've always had automatically are healthy or unhealthy. This is a potent way of taking control.

Now, since you know that the loss of control can have a debilitating effect on your recovery process, and you know you have some ability to determine the amount of control you can exercise over much of your life, you also know a most important fact—*you have to some extent, the ability to affect your recovery.*

Do not underestimate or overestimate this statement. We all have a great deal of control, but we are not omnipotent. None of us is in complete control of the final outcome of any situation, particularly the recovery from cancer. While it behooves cancer patients to muster their every resource to respond to life events in the most positive manner, there is no assurance that the outcome will be as hoped for. But remember, if recovery does not progress as you want it to, it's not because you didn't do enough or didn't do things well enough. Sometimes the outcome is out of our hands.

15. Is there really life after cancer?

❧

Cancer changes many of the day-to-day aspects of living, but life, joy, and involvement can go on during the fight for recovery *if you want and expect them to.* Many people not only live life fully while fighting for recovery but find their enjoyment of life heightened because they learned to "smell the flowers along the way."

Flo Porter, the Wellness Community coordinator who had a double mastectomy and has been cancer-free for six years, says that while she was on a two-weeks-on, two-weeks-off chemotherapy regimen, each two-week period without drugs was among the happiest times of her life.

At the Community we see hundreds of people who, while fighting cancer, are raising children, running businesses, holding down jobs, practicing medicine, falling in or out of love. We see others whose activities are to some extent restricted by the illness but who continue to laugh, read, plan for the future, help other cancer patients, and do many of the things they did before the illness, within their current abilities. On the other hand, if you expect life to be miserable, it will probably be just that.

Michael, who has had a colostomy, was sure he would never again work, love, have friends, or play. Now, almost two years later, he is part of The Wellness Community management, attending meetings several times a month to discuss ways of improving our program. He is also working full-time as an electrician, is planning to be married soon, and his children by his first marriage have moved back with him. All of this is happening while he is still being treated by his medical team and still taking medication.

Michael involved himself in most Patient Active activities, but perhaps the best thing he has done to aid his recovery is his constant interaction with newly diagnosed cancer patients. As he tells his story to others and listens to theirs, faces brighten, stooped shoulders straighten, and eyes start to gleam again—his and theirs. Don't try to tell Michael there isn't life after cancer!

Nancy's story is another dramatic one that reinforces that point. Nancy had breast cancer that had metastasized to the spine. After twenty-four radiation treatments, her physician told her there was nothing more they could do. She recalled:

They told me that my cancer had progressed to such a point that it was time for me to enter a hospice—a place where the process of dying is made as comfortable as possible. As I left for this "final resting place," I took one final look around my home, believing it was the last time I would be in those comfortable, familiar surroundings. It was difficult to say goodbye. But miraculously, after about fourteen weeks in the hospice, I began to improve, and my physicians sent me home and urged me to begin chemotherapy. I had become a hospice graduate.

But, because she had heard so many frightening stories about chemotherapy and was sure it would not do her any good—that she was just going to die anyway—Nancy refused the treatment, despite her husband's urging.

Nancy came to a Sharing Group with her husband, thinking that he would hear so many horror stories about chemotherapy that he would agree with her decision. Then, as she said, "I could die in peace."

Instead, Nancy and her husband heard a variety of reactions to chemo from people who had benefited from it. "What a surprise," she said. "I made up my mind that very night to agree to chemotherapy. From all of the cancer patients I met, I realized that I did not have to die, and with the right attitude, this could be a beginning for me."

One story Nancy heard that night had a major impact on her:

A woman told about coming to The Wellness Community in a walker, and after a few weeks, needing only a cane, and then some time later arriving on her own two feet. Because I had also come in a walker, I dared to make this my goal, too. A few months later, I walked into The Wellness Community with no assistance. No walker, no cane. I had reached my goal.

Today, Nancy is involved in all the activities she did before cancer, but sometimes at a little slower pace.

Of course, whether life is worth living is a matter of individual and personal perception. To one person, life with pain may be well worth fighting for. For another, the inability to do all that she did before the illness may make life intolerable.

As you are reading this, I hope you do not interpret the message to be, "Don't be depressed," or, "Stop crying and get on with your life." These phrases are unrealistic, either as an admonition or as well-intentioned advice. Cancer is bad news. It's something to be worried about. The point here is that there is life after cancer, life worth living, for those who want it, expect it, and work for it.

---

16. I feel that I am to blame for the onset of cancer.

❧

A large precentage of cancer patients who come to us are convinced they are to blame for the development of cancer, but when they meet Patients Active, they are quickly told that they aren't—in fact, couldn't be—to blame. They learn that in order to be at fault for the disease, they would have had to continue acting in a way that could cause cancer after they actually *knew* such actions could have that result. As soon as this subject comes up, they are asked: "Did you, prior to the diagnosis, have the slightest notion that the way you were living and reacting to life events might cause cancer?" Unless the issue is smoking, the answer is invariably no. Only if they *knew* they were risking cancer by some action and did it anyway can they blame themselves.

Smokers who continued to smoke after the Surgeon General's report are the perfect example of taking that kind of risk. They knew that smoking might cause cancer, but they did it anyway. With the possible exception of some foods thought to be carcinogenic, smoking is the only set of circumstances where the threat of cancer is known and the risk taken anyway.

Lynn, the entrepreneur introduced in chapter 5 whose partner squeezed her out of her business, is an example of someone certain she was to blame for the illness. After Lynn was diagnosed as having cancer and started to read about it, she became certain that the trauma of that business upheaval had triggered her disease. She was even more convinced that if she had been in some way better or smarter, she would have done something to prevent the illness. Despite the fact that at the time of the trauma she had absolutely no inkling that her reactions might be making her more vulnerable to cancer, she insisted on blaming herself.

It is possible that the stress of the unpleasant business experience did weaken Lynn's immune system and therefore had some effect on the development of the illness. But if her health was placed in jeopardy by her reactions to her partner's actions, she certainly didn't know it, and she can't be to blame for failing to stop something from happening that she didn't know was happening.

Think back before the diagnosis. Can you remember even one occasion when you thought that the way you were acting might be weakening your immune system? If not, then to blame yourself for the disease is at best unrealistic and at worst dangerous—dangerous because the resulting feelings of inadequacy and guilt may exacerbate your stress.

If you blame yourself, you may trigger two other self-defeating reactions. You may unconsciously forgo taking actions in your fight for recovery, and you may inhibit the spontaneous, self-healing responses your body would automatically take to return to its normal condition.

If you have cancer and blame yourself, this would be a

good time to ask yourself the following questions. Consider each one carefully.

- Do you believe that you are to blame or responsible for the onset of the disease? (If your answer is yes, try to define exactly what you did or didn't do that caused or failed to prevent the disease.)

- Are you sure that different actions on your part would have altered the course of the disease?

- Did you fail to take some action that you, at that time, believed would prevent cancer from developing?

- Finally, the most important question: Did you *know* that the way you were living and coping with the problems of life might be making you more vulnerable to the development of cancer?

I have never known anyone who—even though he blamed himself for the disease—could remember an occasion in which he did or failed to do something while *knowing* such actions might cause cancer (cigarette smoking excepted).

Not long ago, a cancer patient named Linda came to her first Sharing Group and told of participating in a self-help group elsewhere. She had been told, "Unless you are prepared to accept the blame for the onset of the illness, we can't be of much help to you." Several of the people in that self-help session had read some books on the psychosocial aspects of cancer and had misunderstood the authors to say that the acknowledgment of fault was essential for the cancer patient's psychological well-being.

Linda believed they were right and had spent several sessions with that group looking for what she had done wrong. "Then," she said, "we found that what I had done was worry too much about my daughter, who, for about six months, was thought by her doctors to have multiple sclerosis. I shouldn't have worried so much."

Alice, one of the Victors who listened to Linda's story, became incensed. "How in heaven's name," asked Alice, "did you come to the conclusion that you did something wrong because you acted as every mother in the world would? When you were worrying, did you know that worry might cause cancer, and if you had known it, would you have stopped worrying about your daughter? You are not to blame."

Alice then admitted that she, too, had felt self-blame when she was first diagnosed as having cancer. She told Linda:

And I didn't even need a group to help me feel guilty and inadequate. I did it all by myself. You, at least, needed help. When I learned that cancer wasn't my fault, I felt that a massive weight had been taken off my shoulders. The same thing can happen to you. Go back and tell that group they don't know what they're talking about. Tell them nobody except smokers can be to blame for cancer. Ask them what they're doing to make sure they don't get cancer. Tell them if they're so sure the cancer patient must be to blame, they'd better work out a surefire way to ensure that it doesn't happen to them so they don't have to blame themselves later.

When Alice finished, she sat down to ringing applause. We all agreed with her, and when we looked at Linda, she was laughing. She, too, was becoming convinced that self-blame has no place in the cancer patient's life.

17. I feel that I am responsible for not recovering as fast as I think I should.

This conviction is based on the misconception that you are in complete control of the situation and that if you can just do that certain something right, you can cure yourself. To adhere to such a belief, you must be convinced there is a cure that can be effected by doing the right thing the right way. This just isn't so. There is no sure cure for cancer.

Over the years, many people have purported to help cancer patients recover by various psychological or exotic means have told their "patients" that if they have the right attitude or do what is suggested with enough dedication, recovery is "guaranteed." Patients who have setbacks are told, "You must be doing something wrong; aren't you meditating enough?" or "You must not really want to get well." Such statements, of course, are absolute nonsense.

While there are many ways you can participate in your fight for recovery, you don't have the power to ensure recovery. If you believe that recovery is guaranteed if you do it right, any setback will be seen as proof of your inadequacy. *But, no matter what happens, you are not inadequate. What you are doing is right and proper for you.* And just because there is no assurance of winning, you should not stop trying.

If we refused to enter any race we weren't sure of winning, we would enter precious few races. If we didn't take any job unless we were guaranteed of being a great success at it, most of us would always be out of work. Almost nothing in life is certain, and there are very few situations over which we have complete control. The fight for recovery from cancer is not much different from most other efforts we make in life.

For cancer patients, the advice of this chapter is to "go for it" with all your might, with the full realization that just making the effort makes you a winner. Take credit for the successes, but don't assume any blame for the failures. Always be aware that no matter what you have done, you have done all you could, and no one could do it any better.

---

18. If I didn't cause the onset of cancer, how can I affect my recovery?

☙

That question is like asking, "Since I didn't cause the weed to grow, how can I kill it?" If you believe that your actions can influence your immune system, which in turn may alter the course of the disease toward health, what difference does it make whether you caused the illness?

Scientists who have made the investigation of this matter their life's work believe that your participation in the fight for recovery may have a significant and beneficial effect on your recovery process. Those scientists *do not* say that you can help cure yourself *only* if you caused the illness. They *do not* say that if you did not cause the cancer, it's futile to even try to help yourself.

If you fight for recovery, you may enhance the possibility of that recovery, whether or not you were to blame for the development of the disease.

19. I am angry about having cancer. What should I do about that?

☢

Anger, frequently the initial reaction to the diagnosis of cancer, is fraught with risks. No emotion is more likely to suppress the immune system than *unexpressed* anger.

Many experts believe that the inability to express anger is a hallmark of people with cancer. And the problem is made more complex since cancer patients are angry at the fact that they have the illness and don't know at whom to aim that anger.

In most other situations, we can say, "I am angry at him because he was rude to me. She hurt my feelings. He cheated me out of money. She didn't give me the promotion I deserved." But with cancer, that isn't the case (unless you are angry at the environmental polluters or the tobacco companies). There's very rarely anyone to be angry at.

Being angry at someone whom you believe "gave" you cancer has no basis in fact. No one can "give" you cancer. Nor does anger at oneself, even though self-blame is common (see chapter 16). Anger at your physician, which is also unreasonable, will be discussed in chapter 48. And anger at the deity is a matter I'll leave to the theologians.

But the question then is: At whom or what should you be angry because you have cancer? And you might try to think about that question consciously, so that you are not unconsciously being angry at someone or something who doesn't deserve it, and if you find that there is no reasonable object of your anger perhaps it will disappear.

But if the anger remains, keep in mind that it's unwise to ignore or suppress it. A study of women with breast cancer by Martin Abeloff, Ph.D. and Leonard Derogatis, Ph.D., in 1977 found that giving vent to anger was physically beneficial. They wrote, "Women who can express hostility survive metastatic breast cancer longer than non-assertive, compliant women."

In the same vein, Steven Greer, Ph.D., and research assistant Tina Morris in 1979 published a report of a five-year study in which they found that "women who had either a 'fighting spirit' or who were absolute deniers* have a statistically significant advantage both in disease-free interval and mortality compared to those who are hopeless/helpless or stoic acceptors." And it is women who are hopeless, helpless, and stoic who also suppress anger. These relatively recent studies corroborate older studies (by Eugene Blumberg, Ph.D., Philip West, M.D., and Frank Ellis, M.D.,) showing that inhibition of anger is associated with poor prognosis in both men and women with a variety of different cancers.

Patients Active use two general approaches to attacking the problem of irrational anger. You can use either, although we recommend both.

The first is the rational approach—talking about the fury, trying to make some sense of it, and attempting to describe it and explain it to someone. Talking it out forces you to put into coherent form the undisciplined and unbridled emotions running through your mind.

Some people attempting this approach struggle valiantly but are unable to come up with a series of sentences that make any sense. The frustration of that failure sometimes dissolves into laughter or tears, which somehow places the anger in a new perspective. Others describe their anger to cogently and clearly that for the first time they really understand it. And that also dissipates anger.

The second approach to freeing oneself from the ravages of suppressed anger is the screaming method—arranging to be where you can give vent to the fury by screaming, punching pillows, stamping your feet, cursing at the object of your

---

*A *denier* is one who is unable to accept that she has cancer or that the illness has serious implications. Denial is an unconscious psychological reaction; it is not something one can learn. In any event, such a denier is not likely to be reading this book.

hostility, and using every other method of expressing anger you can think of. The purpose is to expel from your body the hostility that is making your life miserable and suppressing your immune system. While this method does not bring about understanding, it certainly releases tension.

There is also a third way of "acting out" anger; unfortunately, it is the most common. In this approach, the cancer patient is not aware he is angry but unconsciously becomes spiteful and antagonistic to everyone around him; the anger leaks out in venom and pettiness. This method doesn't get rid of anything but friends and is in every way counterproductive. The release of tension is so slow that it doesn't do anybody any good. And it occurs when the cancer patient isn't even aware he is angry. Thus, you need always to check within yourself and with friends for this irrational anger and deal with it consciously and directly. You can only benefit.

Finally, anger is not all bad. It can be a powerful motivator. Ask Eddie Foy III, a prominent show business figure and one of The Seven Little Foys. Eddie was diagnosed in 1972 as having malignant melanoma. The cancer was surgically removed, and today he is without symptoms of any kind. When asked on a recent TV program what his initial reaction to the diagnosis was, he responded, "Anger. I was angry then and I'm still angry, and *that anger fueled my drive to get well.*"

Eddie also passed along a George Burns statement he has adopted. When asked how he felt about dying, Burns replied, "I don't want to do it. It's been done."

20. Sometimes I'm ashamed of having cancer, which makes leading a normal social life even more difficult.

❧

The myth that cancer is shameful has existed for a long time and has become part of our culture. Psychiatrist Karl Menninger has characterized cancer as an illness seen by almost everyone as an "evil, invincible predator, not just a disease."

In her book about cancer, *Illness as Metaphor,* Susan Sontag wrote:

> Someone who has had a coronary is at least as likely to die of another one within a few years as someone with cancer is likely to die soon from cancer. But no one thinks of concealing the truth from the cardiac patient. There is nothing shameful about a heart attack. Cancer patients are lied to, not just because the disease is (or is thought to be) a death sentence, but because it is felt to be obscene.

This myth will persist in your mind only as long as you remain isolated from other cancer patients. Soon after they start associating with others with the same illness, most cancer patients lose the feeling of shame and realize that cancer is not obscene and not a curse, but is only a malfunction of the body, just like any other illness.

Cancer patients seem to have difficulty discussing the myth of the "shame" of cancer because it is so unrealistic that they don't know where to start. Does cancer come about because the person was unclean in any way? We know that's not true. Does it affect only poor people and not the rich? Does it develop only in those who are not smart enough?

Does it indicate that the person who develops cancer did things he or she shouldn't have, or failed to do things he or she should? The answer to all these questions is an emphatic no. No one actually knows what causes cancer, and cancer plays no favorites. No one is exempt. Then what is there to be ashamed of?

As unfounded as it is, this myth cannot be ignored or treated like a joke. If it continues, it interferes with social contacts. Just when cancer patients need people the most, their own reclusiveness—and their abandonment by families and friends—somehow seems reasonable. After all, why would anyone want to be with a person who has such a shameful disease? Wouldn't it be awful to impose this shameful disease on friends?

This myth, unlike many others, is easy to get rid of. People quickly learn from other cancer patients how silly it is. Some cancer patients come into Sharing Groups believing that they are proper subjects of scorn, but after meeting others who are dealing with the disease as part of the natural order of things, their attitude quickly changes. I hope that meeting the cancer patients and Victors in this book will have the same effect on you.

If you don't know any other cancer patients, try telling one of your friends that cancer embarrasses you and why. The difficulty of describing the feeling and the basis for it will probably convince you how unfounded the whole idea is.

When cancer patients discard the feelings of shame and embarrassment, they tear down another barrier to living life as it was before the illness. This can quite possibly happen to you.

21. Cancer has changed my appearance so much I don't want to be seen in public.

❧

Almost all cancer patients, at one time or another, experience a change in appearance significant enough to interfere with their normal image of themselves. Very few can just ignore that change and proceed with their daily routine. Many of them want to hide. But hiding is extremely stressful and can hinder the fight for recovery. So it's important to deal with this problem.

It would be easy to accuse anyone who feels uncomfortable about being "different" of acting like a child. But that's not only insensitive but unrealistic. All of us understand the feelings of embarrassment brought about by having a bald head or a large, easily visible scar. We all remember that when we were young, it was uncomfortable to let other kids see us if we weren't dressed exactly as they were, and none of us is that much different now.

But we also know that although it's natural to have that reaction, it's unnecessary and is relatively easy to overcome. You have no idea how many new participants I have watched discard their wigs and "come out of the closet."

These cancer patients meet Victors with similar or worse problems who are living much less inhibited lives because they have already taken the chance of "going public" and have found that people soon accepted them as they were—even without hair or with a scar on their face. Then the newcomer goes out, tests the waters for himself, and has the same experience. When they realize that they don't have to remain out of sight from their friends because of the differences brought about by the illness and its treatment, they enjoy a new sense of freedom.

At your own pace and under circumstances chosen by you—and initially with people you know and trust—test the waters. It takes courage, but it's important to the recovery process.

Ask yourself what you expect to happen when you go public. Will strangers laugh or point at you? Will your friends hide their eyes? Would you react in such an insensitive way if the situation were reversed? What have you got to lose?

True, in the initial contact, you may notice surprise or other emotions in the eyes of your friends. But except in rare situations, that will pass. When it does, the differences between you and the others will not matter, and you will have overcome yet another obstacle on the path to recovery. And, you will have taken back a little more control of your life.

---

22. I feel that my family and friends are abandoning me because I have cancer.

❧

Your observations about your family and friends are probably accurate. But the changes in their behavior are *not* because there is anything wrong with you, and *not* because they love you any less. Most likely it's just that for many people without cancer, it's uncomfortable to be with people with cancer. It's quite possible that you had the same type of reaction to cancer patients before your diagnosis.

This state of affairs has been well documented over the years. Camile Wortman, Ph.D., a noted psychologist who has done extensive work in this field, wrote:

In [one] study of the perceived support available to breast cancer patients, 72 percent of the respondents reported that they were treated differently after people knew they had cancer. Of these, 75 percent indicated that they were misunderstood by others and over 50 percent reported that they were "avoided" or "feared."

Susan Sontag, in her book *Illness as Metaphor,* wrote:

A surprisingly large number of people with cancer find themselves being shunned by relatives and friends and are the object of practices of decontamination by members of their household, as if cancer, like tuberculosis, were an infectious disease. Contact with someone afflicted with the disease regarded as a mysterious malevolency feels (to them) like a trespass.

The myth that cancer is contagious may lead to absurd practices like offering the cancer patient plastic utensils instead of the silverware being used by everyone else at the table.

L. M. Videka, in a report entitled *Psychosocial Adaptations in a Medical Self-Help Group,* wrote:

This general high need of ill people for increased social support comes at a time when those supports are seriously diminished. For example, people with serious illness (especially cancer) are often faced with isolation from friends and family because of fear of contagion, fear of expression of intense emotions or because [the others] don't wish to be reminded of their own vulnerability.

The experience of many Wellness Community participants supports these viewpoints. We have all watched cancer patients becoming more and more isolated simply because they had cancer. But if you have cancer, you don't need this book or any scientific literature to tell you about aloneness. Unless you have very unusual family and friends, isolation is probably part of your own experience.

So, in a way, cancer patients are abandoned, if we understand that word to mean that they are treated differently than they were before the diagnosis. And that abandonment has two aspects, emotional and physical. Some family and friends find the cancer patient's situation so upsetting that they make sure they don't see him or her very often. That's physical abandonment. Others maintain contact, but the relationship becomes strained and the conversations limited to the "right things" they think they are supposed to say; as a result, although the parties are together as much as they were before, the person with cancer has been abandoned emotionally for all intents and purposes.

Family and friends may distance themselves from cancer patients for a number of reasons:

- They can't bear to be with someone they know and love when they feel this person is suffering and ultimately doomed.

- Being with the cancer patient makes them acutely aware of their own vulnerability and their own mortality.

- The only subject they can think about when they are with the person with cancer is the illness, and yet they are absolutely determined that the word "cancer" will never pass their lips when they are with the patient.

- They feel constantly frustrated and inadequate because they want to help and there is nothing they can do.

- They are afraid that cancer is contagious.

- They are afraid the cancer patient will tell them

the truth about how he or she feels, and they are
sure the truth must be horrible.

I am reminded of a statement made by a Wellness Community participant named Stan, who was introduced in chapter 6. "When they ask you how you are, and you answer 'OK,'
that's the end of that conversation," he said. "They really
don't want to know. To people who love you, actually knowing how you feel would be more devastating than they could
bear."

Some of the suggestions in this book can help you break
through the barriers that exist between you and your friends
and family. And it is important to do so, since social contacts
can be such an important part of your recovery process.

---

23. Why do I now find it more difficult to be with people?

℘

That experience is typical and not surprising. Like other cancer patients, you may:

- Remember that before your diagnosis, it was difficult for you to be with people with cancer, and you
"know" that your well friends must find it threatening and unpleasant to be with you now.

- Be frustrated and annoyed that well people can't
understand either the emotional or physical problems you are having.

- Believe that you frighten people because you're
"doomed" in their eyes.

• Be aware that conversation is difficult because you don't know how much others want to hear about the illness, and they're not sure how much you want to tell.

• Believe that because you're wearing a colostomy bag, or are bald from chemotherapy, or are pale and weak, you're so unattractive to others that they don't want to be with you.

• Be actually so weak and incapacitated that you can't participate in life and feel like a dullard.

• Believe that no one would want to be intimate or affectionate with a cancer patient.

When all of the reasons for your reclusiveness are looked at in the cold light of reality, it becomes apparent how much they are based on myths about cancer. That doesn't make them easy to overcome, but it can be done. Chapter 25 and the section of this book on Being a Patient Active will offer suggestions on maintaining contacts with others that can help you in your recovery.

24. Can being alone more than I want to be impede my recovery?

The literature on the subject confirms that aloneness can not only cause depression but may also contribute to illness. If isolation and loneliness can change healthy people into sick ones, those emotions can also retard, if not prevent, recovery from cancer.

A pamphlet published in 1981 by the State of California,

entitled *Friends Can Be Good Medicine,* proclaims, "Friends and other supportive relationships...are as important to your *physical well-being* as they are to your *emotional health.*" The pamphlet adds that "research has shown that there is a correlation between the quality of our relationships and our physical well-being."

The detrimental effect of isolation and forced aloneness upon health was studied by James J. Lynch, M.D., in *The Broken Heart: The Medical Consequences of Loneliness* (1983), using the incidence of heart disease as an example.

Dr. Lynch emphasized the benefits of companionship by comparing the life expectancy of the people of Nevada—who have the shortest life spans in the United States—with that of the people of Utah, who have the nation's longest life expectancy. These adjacent states are quite similar in terms of levels of education, affluence, health consciousness, and physicians per capita.

In other respects the differences between the two states are profound. Unlike many people in Nevada, most people in Utah are extremely religious and neither drink nor smoke. They generally maintain very stable lives. Their marriages are generally secure, family ties remain strong, and most of the state's inhabitants stay in Utah for most of their lives.

Dr. Lynch concluded that people in Utah live longer because they have deeper and longer-lasting relationships—that stable relationships promote health and prolong life. He wrote:

> Human relations are desperately important to both our mental and physical well-being. The fact is that social isolation, the lack of human companionship ...and chronic human loneliness are significant contributors to premature death....Almost every cause of death is significantly influenced by human companionship. Cancer...is signficantly influenced by human companionship....Nature uses many weapons to shorten the lives of lonely people.

Two other studies—the Alameda Study, conducted by Lisa F. Berkman, Ph.D., of Yale University and Lester Breslow, M.D., M.P.H., of UCLA; and the various studies of acculturated Japanese carried out by S. Leonard Syme, Ph.D., and his associates—have also clearly shown that having many social contacts has a beneficial effect on physical well-being.

The Alameda Study took a random sample of some 7000 adults and divided them into age brackets (30 to 49, 50 to 59, and 60 to 69) and levels of social connections. No other criteria—such as weight or smoking and drinking habits— were considered. For the next nine years, the mortality of this group was monitored. In analyzing their statistics, the researchers reached a remarkable set of conclusions: *the more social contacts, the longer the life; the fewer social contacts, the shorter the life*.

For example, the study found that in the 50- to 59-year-old range, for every socially active man who died during the nine-year study, 3.2 men with few social contacts died. For every socially active woman between the ages of 30 to 49 who died, 4.6 socially inactive women died.

The Japanese studies by Dr. Syme also found that close, continuing social contacts have a beneficial effect on health. He compared Japanese men who had come to the United States and had adopted our customs to Japanese men who had remained in Japan or who had come to the U.S. mainland or Hawaii but adhered to their own family-oriented customs. The study found that the group who adopted our custom of greater social isolation suffered heart disease almost three to five times more frequently than did the group who maintained the social ties they had in Japan. Discussing this phenomenon, Dr. Syme wrote:

> The maintenance of close social ties is of paramount value in Japanese culture, as is exemplified by the Japanese saying that "a rolling stone gathers no moss." In the United States, that saying is meant to convey the idea that a person "on the move" is

more highly valued than a person "stuck in a rut."
In Japan, the opposite meaning is intended. In
Japan, moss is a highly treasured plant and a
stone with moss is highly regarded. The only way
one can acquire moss (value) is to remain in the
same place.

The point is that having friends and family around us can,
to some extent, insulate us from illness. Illness flourishes
where aloneness exists. If many and close social contacts are
conducive to a long and healthy life for a well person, they
are indispensable to the cancer patient.

---

25. What should I do about being alone more than I want to be?

క

Unwanted aloneness has two aspects: abandonment on the
part of family and friends, and reclusiveness on the part of the
patient. Both should be attacked.

ABANDONMENT

Abandonment can be physical or emotional, as was explained
in chapter 22. Your friends may stay away from you, or their
reaction to cancer may make conversation so stilted and sterile that they might as well have stayed away.

To ensure that this doesn't happen to you, the most obvious step is to start with your family and friends, and tell
them you need their help. This task may not be easy, but the

reaction you anticipate is probably far worse than the reaction you will actually get. In all likelihood, they are anxious to help.

Do you see what I just did? I slipped in the idea of "asking for help"—and that's just what you should do. Ask your family, friends, and clergy for the kind of help you need.

When you talk to them, make sure the conversation is a two-way street. Ask them how you have changed, and tell them what you want from them. Tell them you would like the relationship to go on much as it had before; or, if you want it to change, tell them how. Discuss your needs with them, and perhaps show them this section of the book to help start the dialogue.

Betty, a Wellness Community participant with ovarian cancer, asked for what she wanted—and got it. Betty was a 45-year-old widow with two sons, 20 and 22, both of whom lived with her. She also had a large group of warm and loyal friends.

When the seriousness of Betty's illness became apparent, her relationship with her sons changed drastically. They stopped discussing with her all of the subjects uppermost in the minds of boys in college, and they no longer brought their friends home. Although her friends made sure she was never alone, they would not talk to her about the illness or their lives. Betty recalled:

> One day, my sons and I began having the same dumb conversations. And I became furious. I yelled and screamed. I told them they were treating me as if I weren't there, and that this was really depressing me. I told them that I was still a part of their lives and they were still a part of mine and that I wanted to be treated that way.
>
> It wasn't a conversation; it was a screaming match. We then all began to laugh and cry, the dam overflowed—and everything changed. They still treat me as if I am sick, because I am. But once

again, I am their mother and they are my sons. I know they love me and want to help me.

After that, it was easy to tell my friends what I thought of the way they were treating me. Some of them understood immediately and changed; some of them just couldn't. But my life is now back to where I look forward to being with people.

Telling your friends and family what you want from them is really all you can do. You can't change anyone but yourself. However, if those close to you don't adopt your suggestions immediately, don't necessarily let that be the end of the effort. For your friends and family, this may be both a difficult and an incomprehensible undertaking. Many people have never had anybody speak to them candidly about their interpersonal wants and desires. In most cases, you are asking them to break a lifelong pattern of privateness and separateness. Many of them have never experienced or contemplated shared intimacy and real, unreserved friendship. So don't be surprised if it takes them some time to respond in the way you want them to.

RECLUSIVENESS

The second phase of the battle against unwanted aloneness is to attack your own reclusiveness. This will require some self-analysis to learn why you now find it more difficult to be with people than you did before the diagnosis. The most difficult part of this exercise will be to be realistic but not too hard on yourself.

Start by asking yourself the following questions:

• Do you actually believe that the people who loved you and enjoyed being with you before the diagnosis don't even like you now? Be very clear here; this question is not about the other people. It's about *you*—what you believe.

If you believe that they are so shallow as to leave at the first sign of adversity—if you believe that you cannot deal with them as you once did, but must now deal with them as strangers or adversaries—then you may have already begun to treat them as strangers and adversaries.

• If the situation were reversed, would you be so upset at their infirmity or physical condition that you would shun them? If your answer is no, why do you believe your friends and family are so much less understanding than you are? Why do you believe that their love and affection is based only on trouble-free times?

Don't sell them short. Assume that they want to continue to be part of your life. And understand that if they are acting strangely, it's because of their fear or lack of knowledge about the illness. Also examine whether your demands on their loyalty and love are reasonable under the circumstances. After all, remember that they have lives independent of yours.

Next, ask yourself and your friends how you have changed since the diagnosis:

• Have you become too demanding?

• Is the illness your only topic of conversation?

• Are you taking advantage of the situation so that others are required to perform tasks that actually are your responsibility?

• Are you forcing others to allow you to act in ways that would otherwise be unacceptable?

• Do you avoid social occasions for realistic reasons, or because of vague, unenunciated fears and expectations of rejection?

- Is your attitude with your friends and family much as it was before the illness, or is it that of consummate victim?

These are questions worthy of careful consideration. So stop now, and reread and think about them. Just understanding the issues, even without fully knowing the answers, can have an effect on the quality of your life, and therefore perhaps an effect on the course of the illness.

A few warnings: When you ask for other people's opinions, listen to what they say, but decide for yourself what's best for you. Don't be surprised if some people fail you; they have problems of their own—fear of facing their own mortality, for example, or the belief that cancer is contagious. And some of them just don't have the time.

Different circumstances spawn different friends. And your circumstances have certainly changed. It's quite possible that your circle of friends will change.

Of course, the mere thought of taking the first step in any of the above suggestions may be enough to make you shudder. But do it anyway. You are a Patient Active. You are joining in the fight to recover. You are replacing decisions based on past experience with actions based on the current situation.

So go to social occasions you would find it easier to avoid. Take part in as many activities as you can. Companionship is part of the battle for recovery, so make sure you have it. One of the happy parts of involving yourself in the fight for recovery is that it doesn't have the same kind of side effects as chemotherapy, radiation, and surgery.

TIPS FOR FAMILY AND FRIENDS

If you have read all the foregoing, you know how important you can be to the cancer patient's fight for recovery.

You can help in two ways. First, when the person with cancer introduces one of the topics discussed here into the conversation, don't be so frightened that you deflect it. Take a chance! It can change your life for the better, too.

Second, when you think the time is right, perhaps you can introduce the subject of how you can help, what is expected of you, or what *you* expect of your relative or friend. All of the suggestions made to the cancer patient also apply to you.

But while using your energy and influence in all reasonable ways to help, you don't have to be a martyr, nor should you take control of the situation. The cancer patient has enough problems with loss of control. As you can see, cancer doesn't present anyone—patient, family, or friends—with easy solutions.

---

26. My family and I don't seem to be relating to one another as we did before my diagnosis.

❧

Cancer in the family always has a profound effect on the entire family structure. This effect can be positive, making the members more aware of how much they mean to each other, or it can place intolerable pressure on the various relationships.

Jimmie C. Holland, M.D., a noted authority on this subject, observed the following in a 1982 interview: "Family members are under enormous stress—sometimes as great as that of the cancer patient himself." Members of the family often have the same feelings of hopelessness/helplessness, passivity, anger, anxiety, and all of the other negative emotions experienced by the cancer patient.

A husband with cancer feels he is no longer of value to the family because he can no longer be the provider. He worries that he is placing a financial burden on the family with the cost of the illness, and that he is not performing his functions as a husband and father. He worries that his children may not turn out well because he can't be the father he thinks he should be, and that his wife may turn to others for the affection to which she is entitled.

The cancer patient also becomes angry and frustrated when his family treats him as they did before the illness: "Don't they know how sick I am?" On the other hand, he becomes just as angry if they treat him as an invalid. He also grows distant from them because he can't tell them how frightened he is: "If they knew, they couldn't handle it." And he pulls away because he can't interact as he once did.

The wife of the cancer patient also has disturbing and guilt-producing thoughts. "What is my life going to be like without him? Can I manage the children and the finances? What are we going to do about all the bills that are running up? How can I continue to be both mother and father to the kids?"

She becomes angry at him, although she knows how irrational that anger is. "Why did he have to go and get sick now?" And she becomes even more angry at herself: "How can I be angry at him and expect him to help share the burdens when he's so sick? A good wife would be worried only about her husband. A part of his illness is probably my fault anyway." She becomes frustrated. She wants so much to help, but there is so little she can do.

Similar feelings arise in the family when it is the wife and mother who has cancer.

If a child is sick, the parents blame themselves. The siblings of ill children also face severe problems. In a 1980 article entitled *Siblings of the Pediatric Cancer Patient,* B. M. Sourkes, Ph.D., reported that one out of two such siblings experienced abdominal pains, trouble in school, and depression. Play and laughter often leave the home. These siblings resent the attention given to their brother or sister, and some-times they mature beyond their years as they help tend the sick child.

So no matter what reaction you are experiencing within the family, it is not abnormal. Troublesome emotions become much less ominous when they are shared, and that means talking about them. Body language, facial expressions, and other subtle ways people use to convey emotions won't do.

The husband of a cancer patient, interviewed as part of a 1985 study by A. Koch, Ph.D., said, "If we love each other, we should know how the other feels without having to express it." He couldn't have been more wrong. No matter how long a couple has lived together, neither really knows what the other is thinking or feeling unless and until told. So the basic rule to help ease the strain on the family brought about by cancer is: communicate.

The need for such communication was clearly demon-strated by a cancer patient named Michelle, whose mother, father, and sister accompanied her to a recent meeting on the topic of "The Family and Cancer." Michelle, 29, lives with her parents. She has had two brain operations. During that meet-ing, tears welled up in her eyes as she described how, since the second operation, she had been terribly afraid that the cancer would recur. She hadn't talked about her fear with her family, she said, because she didn't want them to be fright-ened, too.

Michelle's mother, who was sitting next to her, took Michelle in her arms and they sat there crying and loving. Michelle's father and sister moved closer together and held hands; they didn't want to intrude. Michelle's mother, still not releasing the bear hug on her daughter, said she had always known about Michelle's fear because she and the entire fam-ily were worried about the same thing. "Michelle, we love you," she said. "We are worried about you. But we don't talk to you about it because we don't want you to worry about us."

There—it was out. They loved each other. They were all frightened. And now they could talk about anything. The release and relief they felt was apparent not only on *their* faces, but on the faces of the other twenty-five people in the room.

This story illustrates the wonderful things that can happen when people trust each other enough to be open. If the brother of a cancer patient tells his parents he is worried that they don't love him as much since his brother became ill, they will know he needs more attention. If husband and wife can share their fears of the future, both can bear the burden with greater ease. It doesn't make sense to hide from family members what they probably know already.

Communication with people other than family members can also be helpful. Consider Cindy, for instance, whose husband had lung cancer. Not long ago, a newspaper reporter asked her what her reaction had been when she heard her husband had cancer. She replied:

> I felt like life was over for me. Yet although I am not of the Norman Cousins mold, I knew I was going to fight. At home, I am the "earth mother" to my husband and children, and although we discuss our mutual fears, I try to be strong most of the time. So I need other people to give me strength to go back to the battleground. When I cry and show my fear to my friends, that releases the tension.

As Cindy's answer shows, it is very helpful if, as a concerned family member, you can talk frankly and openly about your fears and worries to someone who is relatively objective. A support group of a special friend can play that role, or you might turn to a therapist.

A caveat is in order here. Cindy encountered the following when she looked for a therapist:

> The first thing I did was quite healthy. I went to three different therapists, but none of them felt equipped to help me. Each looked for someone else who was more used to counseling people in my

situation. They couldn't handle me because they
wanted to "fix" me, and they couldn't accept my
pain and fear.

So when you pick the special friend or a therapist, make
sure they know what you want and need. Tell them you're not
looking to be "fixed" or necessarily advised—rather, what you
want is someone who will listen, understand, and be your
friend and help you translate the irrational into the rational.

One family devised its own approach to opening up communication. Several nights a week after dinner, everyone who
was home would sit together for a short time and tell some
of the happy or worthwhile events that had happened that
day, and they kept a family journal. This simple device, they
said, somehow kept the family together. It sounds like a good
idea to me.

---

27. I sometimes feel that I just want to give up—that fighting to recover is too hard and is taking too long.

❧

Fighting for one's own recovery is not easy. It's hard and constant work. Sooner or later, almost every cancer patient seriously wonders, either consciously or unconsciously, whether
it's worth it. Why not just give up?

Although some of your well friends might be horrified by
such an attitude, a support group at The Wellness Community
would understand and applaud the fact that you have brought
the question to consciousness, because the answer may have
serious implications. Cancer patients can drift into a giving-
up attitude without realizing it.

The most important lesson you can learn from this chapter is to make sure this is not happening to you. Ask yourself if you might unconsciously be giving up. If you're not sure, ask yourself the following questions. Although some may seem to have obvious answers, the responses are often other than you would expect.

• Was life before the diagnosis worth living? If it was not, it will be difficult to keep fighting to return to that life unless you now know how to make it better.

• Do you believe there is a possibility that you will recover? If you don't, it is difficult to keep fighting a battle you're convinced you will lose.

• Is there anything you can do to aid the recovery process?

• Is there still room for joy and involvement in your life?

• Are you sure those reasons actually apply to you?

• Would life as an ex-cancer patient with the results of the illness be acceptable to you?

At this point it might be wise to read the remarks made by Michael B. Van Scoy-Mosher, M.D., a prominent Los Angeles oncologist, when we asked him whether he believes that the participation of a cancer patient in the fight for recovery can have any effect on that recovery process.

The question I ask myself is, Do all of us, or any of us, have the power within us to control cancer—to make it reverse or at least intensify the effects of medical therapy? Of course, no one really knows whether we do or not, but my belief is that many of us do. The problem is working out some way to harness that power in each situation. And I suspect that certain individuals have been able to do that, and this accounts for some very surprising results in relation to cancer.

The thing I've been struck by, not all the time but reasonably consistently, is that the people who seem to do the best with cancer—whether that means "cured" or "complete remission" with good control of the disease for a significant amount of time—have certain abilities. One of them is that cancer doesn't dominate all of their life. They don't become obsessed with it. They are able to go on with a lot of the other parts of their life and periodically put the cancer in the background.

The reason that people are obsessed with cancer is that they feel it's uncontrollable, that they can't possibly do anything about it, and that the treatment won't help. But if they are aware of the possibility that they can control it, then they can afford the luxury of spending some time in the day not thinking about it.

The first step, and I tell all of my patients this, is that they have to develop a feeling that they can beat it and control it. Not that they are necessarily going to, but that there is the possibility that they can. (Emphasis added.)

I believe that some people intuitively know there is such a possibility. Other people need that belief implanted in their minds. Everyone needs it encouraged and reinforced.

What I want my patients to focus on is getting well and what they can do about it, rather than to focus on the cancer and how to be sick. Your program [The Wellness Community] focuses on getting well...you focus on hope rather than acceptance. Teaching people how to accept their impending doom or that they're going to be sick for the rest of their lives focuses on the wrong thing and nurtures and reinforces the wrong concepts. I want my patients to learn how to get well. It's not always going to work despite the best of everybody's efforts. It's not always going to work, by any means.

Also, I've noticed that there are some people whose illness, personality, and life situation are of such a nature that no matter what kind of treatment they get, and no matter what they do, they're going to get well. There are, of course, other people about whom the opposite is true. Then there is a group in the middle who could go either way. And that's where The Wellness Community program and my best efforts can make the difference.

From my point of view, the very best kind of patient is the patient who understands the treatment, the need for it, and the side effects so it is not some mysterious thing forced on him. That kind of patient is therefore under a lot less strain, because he doesn't feel like he is being pushed around. And that makes life a lot easier for me. Very often, oncologists are placed under tension because we seem to be trying to talk our patients into doing something they don't want to do. With the understanding patient, there is an adult-to-adult relationship. We both know that we are there not to fight each other. We are there to fight the cancer.

Also, keep in mind that no one should fight to recover just because someone else wants him to. In her book *On Death and Dying,* Elisabeth Kubler-Ross, M.D., a noted thanatologist (one who studies death and dying), advised the friends and family of very sick people thus: "If the patient's wishes are contrary to our beliefs and convictions, we should express this conflict openly and leave the decision up to the patient as far as further treatments are concerned." At The Wellness Community, when an individual chooses to give up the fight, after a discussion with the members of his group, they support him in that decision.

But always remember that continuing to fight for recovery can have some wonderful benefits that just may enhance the possibility of recovery.

---

28. What are the signs that I have unconsciously given up?

இ

If you find yourself resisting the suggestions in this book, perhaps now is the time to figure out why. To begin, let's examine how you are reacting to a suggestion that's easy to follow: to be more careful with your diet. If you find that you're still eating everything you ate in the past, despite knowing that some of it is not good for you, you might ask yourself the following: Is having something taste good in your mouth that important? Or is getting well that unimportant?

Could it be that you want to eat what tastes good—and the hell with control and nutrition—because you unconsciously believe you don't have much time left and there isn't much other joy in life anyway? These are important questions that boil down to one specific issue: Have you unconsciously given up?

Smoking is another sign of surrender. Cancer patients know, often better than anyone else, that smoking is harmful. And yet many of them persist in puffing away. The only rules of The Wellness Community are "No smoking and all other rules of common courtesy." Yet there are participants—people who say they want to be Patients Active—who take a break from whatever they're doing to "grab a smoke."

These smokers seem to be making the following state-ment: "I'll take as much pleasure as I can because I really don't have many left and precious little time to enjoy the few I have." But that's not a healthy attitude. That's a definite sign of little hope. And without hope, the chances of recovery are not as great as they might otherwise be.

Keep in mind that there's nothing wrong with giving up if it's done *consciously*. But if one part of you wants to fight to get well, and another is shouting that nothing you can do will make any difference and you might as well enjoy what's left, you must recognize the conflict and decide which course you want to follow.

That decision may be the most important you have ever made. By deciding to fight, you could be sending a message to your body countermanding your previous unconscious orders to give up. You might also find yourself energizing a new and better way of dealing with the illness—better compliance with medical advice and more activity as a Patient Active, both of which can only be helpful.

---

29. In what way can the pursuit of happiness be a part of my fight for recovery?

❧

This short chapter summarizes the entire message of this book to the effect that *the pursuit of happiness should be an integral part of the fight for recovery*, just as chemotherapy, radiation, and surgery are often components of the same fight.

A MORE SCIENTIFIC WAY OF SAYING THAT THE PURSUIT OF HAPPINESS SHOULD BE A PART OF THE FIGHT FOR RECOVERY

• Most unremitting, long-term stress—negative emotions, unhappiness—depresses the immune system, the body's first line of defense against cancer.

• It is hypothesized that positive emotions—happiness—strengthen the immune system.

• A depressed immune system can impede the fight for recovery. A strengthened immune system may make the possibility of recovery more likely.

• Therefore, the pursuit of happiness, if for no other reason than to bolster the immune system, should be a part of the fight for recovery.

III
BEING A PATIENT ACTIVE

30. How can I maximize the possibility that my emotions will strengthen my immune system?

❧

We know that the fight-or-flight response suppresses the immune system, which is the body's first line of defense against cancer. So the purpose of this chapter is to help you discover if you have any habitual methods of reacting to life's problems that keep you in a prolonged, unremitting fight-or-flight reaction, and if you do, to help you learn ways of modifying or changing them.

In chapter 2, we discussed the chain of events that leads to suppression of the immune system, including the three points at which positive action can be taken to head off a fight-or-flight response (see diagram on page 14). In this chapter, we will concentrate on attempting to forestall the fight-or-flight response at the first of these points, the stressor. In chapter 31, we'll discuss aborting this response at the point of the stress. In chapter 32, we'll consider a method of intervening at the final stage, between the stress and the fight-or-flight response.

As you may recall, a stressor is any event we perceive that evokes an emotional response. Stress is the mental reaction to becoming aware of the stressor, while the physical adaptation to the stress is the immune-suppressing fight-or-flight response. (For an elaboration of these concepts, see chapter 2.)

In this chapter, we will consider only those long-term, unremitting stressors that require changes in coping styles—that is, psychological changes. We will not consider stressors that can be dealt with in a pragmatic way, such as by leaving an overly stressful job; nor will we consider short-term stressors, such as making a speech before a large audience, because they are not among the factors that lead to developing cancer.

The experience of a patient named Nadine illustrates the interruption of the immune-suppressing chain of events at the point of the stressor. In a discussion with other cancer patients, Nadine realized she had been a "doormat" for her husband and two children for the twelve years of their marriage—that what *they* wanted always took priority over what she wanted.

Much more importantly, Nadine discovered that a part of her was constantly angry at her family's insensitivity to her needs. She had never discussed that anger with anyone.

By recognizing that she was constantly angry and that the cause of her anger was her family's insensitivity to her needs (the stressor), Nadine had taken the first step toward heading off the fight-or-flight reaction.

The next step was to find a way to eliminate that stressor, and there are two methods she could use to do that: Do what she could to make sure the stressor did not recur, or, if that didn't work, use the "act as if" method.

Nadine tried the first method. She told her husband and children of her anger and asked them to be more considerate of her needs and desires. They tried, but, because of inertia and habit, not much changed. And after several months Nadine saw that the first option had failed.

Nadine's next step was to "act as if" standing up for her own self-interest was what she felt like doing.

The "act as if" technique is based on the concept that in most situations, we are presented with two options: we can react either *reflexively* or we can react *rationally*. Most of the time, most people react reflexively—automatically, never considering their alternatives. Usually that's not harmful, because most decisions are inconsequential. However, when those reflexive reactions provoke constant negative emotions (as they did in Nadine's case), it becomes essential, particularly for the cancer patient, to consider a more deliberate and healthier way of reacting—namely by doing what she believes is best for her "as if" that's what she feels like doing and always considering her alternatives.

Nadine had always reacted to every demand from her family with a "Yes, dear." Whenever her son wanted a ride, she complied, no matter what her own plans were. When she was invited to attend a function she would have enjoyed, she always refused the invitation if it would keep her from preparing the dinner her family expected. Because of her training and background, it had never occurred to her that a "good" wife and mother had any alternative.

After a dozen years of marriage and a lifetime of compliance, "acting as if" her own needs and pleasures were important was a difficult change for Nadine. It was made even harder because her family unconsciously resisted her efforts. She was often tempted to give in. However, she persevered, "acting as if" assertiveness and reasonable self-interest were natural for her—"as if" she were a wife and mother, not a maid and chauffeur.

Here is how Nadine handled situations as they arose: First, she would recognize the stressor—for instance, a request for her to do something for her family. That recognition alone was a major step in the right direction and a boost to her morale. After identifying the problem, she would consider the request; if it was reasonable, she would comply.

However, if the request was unreasonable, even though she felt like saying yes out of habit, she would "act as if" she felt like saying no. She would refuse the request or suggest an alternative. For example: "How would it be if I went to my meeting first and took you to your friend's house later?" Eventually, considering her own desires as well as those of others became Nadine's natural reaction. In the process, her anger started to subside, taking some of the pressure off her immune system.

If an individual "acts as if" long enough and consistently enough, soon his new way of responding will be the way he naturally *feels* like acting. And if this releases a cancer patient from a consistently negative reaction to a life event, that may be a momentous step in the right direction.

I hasten to add that choosing what is best for you can be, and often is, based on feelings of love, charity, and compassion. No one is suggesting hedonism.

After a while, Nadine's family started to understand her new position, and their unreasonable requests became less and less frequent. Certainly, Nadine took a risk that her family would become completely alienated and that she would then be faced with returning to her old ways or making a new life for herself. Luckily, Nadine never had to make that choice. The whole family benefited from her newfound assertiveness. Currently, Nadine is doing quite well in her fight against cancer.

Take a moment to examine your own life—either with a group, with a friend, or alone—to see if you can detect any constantly recurring stressor. This can be a difficult assignment. It took Nadine quite a while to admit to herself that she resented her family's insensitivity to her needs. But once she did, it presented her with the opportunity to actively decide what action she wanted to take, instead of reacting reflexively. What a wonderful feeling of freedom and power.

After becoming aware of a stressor, see if you can eliminate it in some pragmatic way. If that can't be done, decide how it would be best for you to react to that stressor, and then "act as if" that is the way you feel like reacting. If you keep it up long enough, you may be amazed by the results. It's not always easy, it takes perseverence, and it doesn't always work. But it's part of your fight for recovery, and thus is worth the time and effort. And remember, if it doesn't work for you, that doesn't mean you didn't do it right. It only means it didn't work.

31. If situations that invariably invoke a negative reaction are unavoidable, how can I minimize the physical harm that may result?

❧

The previous chapter concerned itself with interrupting the chain of events leading to the fight-or-flight response at the point of the stressor (see diagram on page 12). This chapter will consider interrupting that chain at the point of the stress. Generally, this can be done by making sure that the reaction to the stressor is as mild as possible, because the less dramatic the reaction, the less intense the fight-or-flight reaction— and therefore the less severe the suppression of the immune system.

Charlene is a good example of someone who substituted a mild reaction for what had been a rather violent one. A 32-year-old married woman and an officer of a large corporation, Charlene had Hodgkin's disease. Her co-worker Jeff was rude to her and interrupted her constantly, which infuriated her. After she did everything she could to persuade Jeff to be more polite, all to no avail, she decided that since she could not change him, she would change the way she reacted to him. Realizing that Jeff wasn't in the way of getting the job done but was just an annoyance, she soon saw him as a buffoon and a fool rather than a dangerous foe. In the process, her anger turned into amusement. (This process was not as easy as it sounds.)

Then there's Leslie, a 52-year-old single woman with breast cancer, who has a job she can't afford to quit because of the medical insurance it provides. The job, however, includes a domineering and very unpleasant supervisor. Many nights, Leslie went home with her stomach in knots because of the supervisor.

With her friends, Leslie decided that since she couldn't change her supervisor, she would change her reaction. She would see herself not as a weak and helpless child being bullied by an all-powerful persecutor, but rather as an adult whose job required her to interact with an unpleasant superior. Before, Leslie had felt that she was walking into a combat zone every morning. But now she recognized that, like almost everyone else in the world, she had a job that included some aspects not to her liking. This has not been an easy adjustment for Leslie to make, but she is working on it day by day.

Keep in mind that it's not possible or even desirable to change every negative emotion into a positive one. Sometimes it's reasonable to feel disagreeable emotions such as fear, guilt, or anxiety. The question then is, Now that you know it's best for you to keep your reaction to a stressor as bland as possible, how do you do it?

An important first step is to determine whether your stress is realistic, appropriate, and based on current, not remembered, facts. If it is—and it well might be—there is no reason and no way to change it. *On the other hand, if you become aware that your reaction to a particular stressor is neither realistic, appropriate, nor based on current facts, the reaction will automatically disappear without any effort on your part, to be replaced by a more realistic and appropriate response. It's just not possible to continue to react to a problem in an unrealistic or inappropriate way once you know that such a reaction is based on something other than current reality.* I know this is hard to believe, but read on.

If you see an uncaged tiger, it's realistic to be afraid it will bite you. However, when you are sure that the tiger has been drugged and has neither teeth nor claws, that fear will disappear. And that's just the point. If you are afraid or worried about something you believe can hurt you, that fear will vanish when you find out that (a) it *can't* hurt you; (b) that the hurt cannot be severe; or (c) that it is very unlikely to happen.

To determine whether your reaction to a particular

stressor is realistic and appropriate, start by describing the stressor to yourself, to a friend, or to a group, being as objective as possible. Tell them, for instance, how ever since your divorce, every relationship you've been in has been a stressor because you're sure, now more than ever, that you're unlovable and destined to spend the rest of your life alone. Or tell them that ever since your promotion, your job has been a huge stressor because you're sure you're not good enough to do the work.

When you do this, go into detail and be specific, but omit any drama and pathos; concentrate on the stressor. Don't let your emotions confuse the issue. Ask yourself and your group the questions set out below. If you are impersonal and stick to it long enough, the answers to these and other pertinent questions will quite likely become apparent.

1. What do you really fear? That question is often very difficult to answer, although the answer may seem obvious at first. Consider the mother who wanted her son to become a brain surgeon like his father, and was "worried sick" (notice the phrase "worried *sick*") because he was dropping out of school to become a wood-carver. When asked why she was so anxious to have her son follow in his father's footsteps, she replied that she wanted him to be happy. We know, and she knew, that it's quite possible he would have been miserable as a physician and happy as a wood-carver. So what was it she really was afraid of? The possibilities are endless and cry out for examination.

2. Do you have reason, based on current events, to believe that what you are afraid of is likely to happen, or are you basing your concern on past events? A perfect example is Jenny, who expected that every man would leave her, because when she was a child, her father left her for two weeks every month in his job as a traveling salesman.

3. If what you are worried about takes place, how badly will you be hurt, if at all? If you believe you need that man (or woman), as the song says, more than life itself, you will always be afraid of being left and that life will no longer be worth living. But when you learn that you don't *need* that person but only *want* her (or him), and that life will go on even without this person—it always does—the fear changes to something much less drastic.

4. How likely is it that what you are worried about will take place? It's unrealistic, for example, for a student who has always received all A's to worry about flunking out.

Still other questions (and you can probably think of more):

- Are you overreacting?
- Is there a more reasonable way for you to react?
- Is your reaction reasonable and rational?

Embarking on this quest for clarity will take work, patience, courage, and a willingness to hear observations that may often surprise and sometimes distress you. But learning that your anxiety is unrealistic and hard on your immune system may be an important step on your road to recovery.

32. What is directed visualization and how can I use it in my fight for recovery?

❧

In the two preceding chapters, we discussed interrupting the chain of events leading to the fight-or-flight response at the point of the stressor and the stress (see diagram on page 12). This chapter will suggest how you can intervenes between the stress and the unhealthy fight-or-flight reaction.

Suppose Frank is the owner of a business that's been on the verge of bankruptcy for the last three years, and if he's going to be able to save it at all, it will take three more years of hard work. He knows that if he makes one mistake, that's the end of his business.

Frank has an unchangeable stressor to which his reaction is appropriate, and unless he does something about it—intervenes between the stress and the body's adaptation to it—his body is going to be in the immune-suppressing fight-or-flight mode for the next three years.

The technique that we at The Wellness Community suggest to intervene between the stress and fight-or-flight reaction is called *directed visualization,* a combination of meditation and guided imagery. Meditation is described in *The Relaxation Response,* by cardiologist Herbert Benson, M.D. Guided imagery is explained in *Getting Well Again,* by O. Carl Simonton, M.D., an oncological radiologist, and Stephanie Matthews-Simonton. Although both components of directed visualization are discussed in this chapter, if you want more information, I highly recommend both books.

When most people hear words like *meditate* or *directed visualization,* they immediately picture a yogi sitting in the lotus position in a dimly lit, incense-filled room. Furthermore, they assume that the yogi must have great knowledge, must have suffered and studied extensively and devoted his life to this practice.

But the technique suggested here has no connection with religion, mysticism, the occult, or the exotic. It is an effective, pragmatic method of relaxation that can have a significant beneficial effect on the immune system. It does not take any great skill, practice, or knowledge. Anyone can do it, and there is no way you can do it wrong. No matter how you perform it, it will have some beneficial effect on your immune system. Finally, be assured that once you generally understand the purpose and the simple method described here, there is nothing more anyone can teach you that you won't learn just by continuing to meditate.

Just because this technique is easy and not terribly time-consuming, don't be fooled into believing it's not worth doing. Many Patients Active consider directed visualization one of the key elements of their fight for recovery. One participant, in describing his bout with cancer, said:

> I also involved myself in directed visualization. I really think it's critical. I did it twice a day for a year. And if you ask me whether I believe the mind has power over the body to cure things that are wrong with it, I would tell you that I do. And whether it does or doesn't is almost irrelevant. I thought it was helping me, so I felt good about it. I felt I was in control—that I was going to be victorious.
>
> I think people with cancer who don't visualize are missing the boat, because visualization costs nothing, has no bad side effects, and it makes you feel good even if it doesn't cure cancer—which it might. I don't understand people who don't use every tool available.

The full text of the twenty-minute directed visualization technique we recommend is printed in chapter 33. As you'll see, the first ten minutes are devoted to meditation for the purpose of eliciting the Relaxation Response; the second ten minutes are devoted to guided imagery, which is an attempt to enhance the immune system and "aim" it at the cancer. You can read the text onto a tape and play it back as required.

HOW MEDITATION WORKS

As you've already learned, when we perceive an unpleasant stressor, the brain releases a flood of hormones that prepare the body for action. Since the flow of these hormones can be physically harmful if continued for too long, a method had to be found to turn off this flood.

Dr. Benson discovered that meditation accomplishes this goal. He named the body's reaction to meditation the Relaxation Response. *During this process, every aspect of the fight-or-flight response is reversed, and the immune system regains the strength it had prior to the perception of the stressor.* No side effects have been noted among people who utilize this approach no more than twice daily for twenty minutes at a time.

HOW GUIDED IMAGERY WORKS

The guided imagery half of directed visualization is an attempt to enhance the power of the immune system and "aim" it at the cancer through visualization.* The Simontons, the originators of guided imagery for cancer patients, were aware of studies showing that people could exert substantial control over internal physical functions once thought to be outside conscious control (such as blood pressure, heart rate, and skin temperature) by using visualization. They hypothesized that with the same technique, people could direct the im-

---

*As used here, visualization involves imagining a particular situation with the intention that such envisioning will effect a specific result in your body. For example, you imagine your arm in a bucket of ice water, hoping that your skin temperature will fall (see chapter 4 on biofeedback).

mune system, one of the internal bodily functions thought to be automatic, to become stronger, concentrate its efforts on the cancer, and perhaps alter the course of the disease toward health.

In their book, the Simontons describe how their first subject was told to enter into the process by relaxing his body and picturing himself in a pleasant, quiet place, such as a stream or under a tree. He was then told to:

> ... imagine his cancer vividly, in whatever form it seemed to take. Next, Carl asked him to picture his treatment, radiation therapy, as consisting of millions of tiny bullets of energy that would hit all the cells, normal and cancerous, in their path. Because the cancer cells were weaker and more confused than normal cells, they would not be able to repair the damage. Carl suggested that the normal cells would remain healthy while the cancer cells would die. Carl then asked the patient to form a mental picture of the last and most important step—his body's white blood cells coming in and swarming over the dead cancer cells and flushing them out of his body. In his mind's eye, he was to visualize his cancer decreasing in size and his health returning to normal. After he completed the exercise, three times a day, he was to go about whatever he had to do for the rest of the day.

The Simontons reported the remarkable recovery of this first patient, as well as several other case histories with various degrees of happy endings. Although their work has caused some controversy, their procedure is now widely used in many traditional medical establishments as an adjunct to conventional treatment.

Certainly no one as yet knows whether directed visualization works to reduce the size of a tumor or enhance the possibility of recovery. However, we do know that it makes people feel better, brings about the Relaxation Response, sometimes reduces pain, and returns some control over life to the individuals who practice it.

People who are very much involved in fighting for recovery take to this device extremely well, experiencing a feeling of participation in the fight for recovery, with the certainty that it has some beneficial physical results.

---

33. Script for directed visualization

❧

PROCEDURE FOR LISTENING TO DIRECTED VISUALIZATION

- **Allot about twenty minutes twice a day.**
- **Sit quietly where you can be alone and quiet for that period of time.**
- **Play the tape. It contains all the directions.**
- **Make a conscious effort to follow the directions.**

This script should be read slowly and deliberately into a tape recorder in your normal voice. Pause periodically so that when you listen to the tape, you will have time to absorb the instructions.

This is going to be a time of complete relaxation...a conscious effort to relax as completely as possible. Get into as comfortable a position as you can, and close your eyes. For the next couple minutes, just concentrate on your breathing.

To the best of your ability, see your lungs...see how they

feel, consciously see how they feel while they're completely
expanded, and see how they feel after you exhale. Be aware
that there's no right way and no wrong way to do what you're
doing now... that whatever results you get are perfect results,
and that if all you do is relax, that's wonderful. This is not a
time to be worrying about any of the things that are happening in your day-to-day life. This is a time only for you, and you
can let it all hang out. For this very short period of time, you
can completely relax. You are never out of control. You can
feel completely secure.

Now, once again, concentrate on your lungs. Picture
them in your mind's eye. See if you can see them filled... see
if you can see them after you relax. And if your mind drifts
away, and you want to, just bring it slowly back to where you
are or where you want it to be. You're doing nothing wrong,
and anything you do will be a success. And if you hear my
voice, that'll be fine... and if you don't, that's fine, too. You
can be absolutely sure that your subconscious is hearing
every word I say.

And now, perhaps, in your mind's eye—way, way out in
space—you can see a word all lit up... and the word is
RELAX. Just relax... and now that same word is about a foot
in front of your forehead... just see it about a foot in front of
your forehead, the word RELAX. And now inside your forehead, see that word, and just relax.

Now perhaps, if you want to, pay attention to your left
foot, and the toes on your left foot, and your ankle, and let
them all relax... and all the cares and tensions of the day just
drain down into the floor. Consciously let them relax... and
any noise you hear will only serve to deepen your relaxation.

And now pay attention, if you will, to your right shoulder.
All the muscles of your right shoulder, completely relaxed. All
the cares of the day drain away and leave you. And consciously check your right shoulder to see if there's any tension there. Think about it. And now all of the muscles and
tendons of your right foot, and the toes of your right foot, and
the ankle, just let them relax. And now the calf of your right

leg, let it relax. And for this very short period of time in your mind's eye, perhaps you can see that wonderfully long bone running from your ankle to your knee in your right leg...See how wonderfully straight and long and solid it is...and what a wonderful feat of construction. Let it relax...let all the muscles just relax...and the muscles of your left calf...relax. And way, way out in the future, and way, way into the past.

And this is a learning process...just like when you were a very, very little person and you didn't know how to ride a bicycle, or tell time, or read. And when you were out learning to ride a bicycle, you couldn't even tell how long you were out there because you couldn't tell time, and you didn't know whether there was a difference between writing and printing ...and this is also a learning process...learning to relax... learning to be at ease.

And now let all the muscles of your left shoulder completely relax...Let it just droop toward the ground...and rest comfortably against the seat you're in. Let it relax. And now the muscles of your stomach. Let your stomach just hang out...just relaxed. Once again, it's like when you were a very, very little person, just learning how to do all of the things you had to do, like telling time and reading...And now the muscles of your left thigh...This is a time for relaxation...and you don't have to go to sleep...but if you do, that's fine... and if my voice drifts away, that's fine...and if your mind drifts away, that's fine, too. Whatever you do is wonderful. Completely relax.

And now all the muscles of the right thigh...just let them relax. All the tensions of the day just drain out of them into the seat below you. And there's that word RELAX. Consciously in your mind is the word RELAX, way, way out in the past...just in the past...and right behind your forehead.

And all the muscles of your face now...the muscles of your lips, your cheeks, and your forehead, just let them fall toward the ground and your stomach. And your chest...once again, your chest just relaxed, and now your back, and your complete right arm and the fingers of your right hand. And if there's any part of your body that's not completely relaxed already, it soon will be.

You may be surprised to see how relaxed you are already. That may come as a surprise to you...and as I said, if there's any part of your body that's not yet relaxed, it soon will be. And if there's any part of your body that's not feeling as comfortable as it might, concentrate on that part of the body for the next few seconds...just think of it...and send all the endorphins* of the brain down in that area. Consciously be aware of any part of your body that's not as comfortable as it might be.

And now all the muscles and sinews and tendons of your left arm and your left hand and the fingers of your left hand completely relax. And all the muscles of your neck and your shoulders and your chest and your buttocks and the whole pelvic area now...Think about the whole pelvic area...once again your face...and your head...And if my voice drifts away, that's fine, just as long as you're sitting back comfortably and relaxing.

Many things are changing in your body, all of which are normal and wonderful, just through your relaxation.

And now, perhaps, if you want to, you'll see yourself at the top of a flight of ten steps going down. You've been at the top of stairs before, and you will be again. So this is completely familiar to you. This is a time when you can just put your trust in the world. You will never be out of control in any way. You can trust...like you did when you were a very, very little person. And everything is going to turn out exactly as you want it to. We're going to walk down these steps together, if you want to, and with every step down you take, you're going to relax just a little bit more.

And now, if you will, you can take the first step down... and you've taken one step down, and you have nine to go. And with every step down, you relax just a little bit more. And any noise you hear will serve to relax you just a little bit more.

*Endorphins are pain-killing chemicals that occur naturally in the brain.

And way, way out in the future, and way, way back in the past, and right behind your forehead is that word RELAX.

And now, you take another step down. And with every step down you relax just a little bit more, and now you've taken two steps down, and you have eight steps to go... And take another step down... relaxing just a little bit more with every step you go down. And feel that relaxation in your body... and you may be surprised at how relaxed you feel already. And now take another step down, and that's four steps down, and you have six to go. This is a time for relaxation. It's not necessary for you to go to sleep, but if you want to, that's fine. If it happens, that's fine; or if your mind drifts away, that's fine. Nothing that you do is wrong.

Take one more step down. And now you're halfway down the stairs... You have five more steps to go... and you take another step down. And see yourself, consciously see yourself, on the sixth step down, and how comfortable you feel, and how secure you feel, and how trusting you feel. And now another step down... and now you've taken seven steps down and you have three to go. And there's that word RELAX shining way, way out in the heavens and behind your forehead at the same time... and you take another step down... and you've taken eight steps and you have two more to go. And now one more step... and you've taken nine steps down and you have one to go... and now take that last step down, and you're all the way down to the bottom of the stairs. And you may be surprised at how relaxed you really are.

And now, if you want to, and it's easy for you to do... perhaps you can see yourself on a lovely, lovely, warm, comfortable beach. And way out in front of you is a calm, calm, very blue ocean. Very calm and very blue. And see if you can smell what the ocean smells like. Really try to smell it. Be there. And the sun is just beating down on your body in a way that can't hurt you under any circumstances... and feel the cool breeze over your body and how comfortable that feels. And hear the ocean lapping on the shore. Listen to what it sounds like. And underneath your feet is the warm sand, just the right temperature, the way you like it best. And behind you is an enormous beach, friendly and protective and just wonderful.

And now, while you're standing there, perhaps you can see yourself as a very, very little person at a time when you were very happy, very content, and very secure. And feel that happiness, and feel that security, and feel that carefree feeling, and know that that's you... And remember that any noise you hear will just relax you further. And you can call back this feeling of happiness and contentment any time you want to... it's *your* feeling and it's *your* memory. The only one in the world who has that memory is you.

And now, if you want to, see yourself standing on the beach once again, as an adult... And now, if you want to, knowing that there's a large, comfortable beach towel on the beach to guard your head, see yourself lie down on your back and feel how secure the ground is under you, holding your calves and your backside and your shoulders and your head. Feel how secure that is.

And now, perhaps you'll see yourself surrounded by a lovely golden light. It covers every inch of your body while all the normal functions go on... you breathe very normally and your pores are open, and every normal function goes on. And that lovely, lovely golden light is a combination of all of the healing power of the universe, and all of the healing power of your own body, and all of the healing power of any medication you're taking or radiation you're receiving, or anything you're taking... and that golden light can go anyplace you tell it to.

And now, if you want to, see that part of your body that is not exactly as you want it to be. And direct that golden light to go to that part of your body and surround that area or areas. And know that the golden light surrounding the part of your body that is not as healthy as you want it to be, combines all of the healing power of the universe, and all of the healing power of your body, and all of the healing power of any medication that you're taking. It's an extraordinarily powerful elixir. And any cancer cells that are there are weak and erratic cells and easily defeated. And you can tell the golden light to crush any cancer cells, and to diminish any tumor . . . and to do anything you want it to do . . . and it's a powerful, vital, vigorous force and the cancer cells are weak and erratic.

Consciously see the golden light surrounding all of the area where your body is not in the condition you want it to be. And notice . . . notice how it can bring the endorphins of your brain down into that area and soothe any pain . . . and help to alleviate any problem that's going on in your body. And tell that golden light to do what you want it to do. It is *your* golden light. It is going to go where you want it to go. And by telling it where you want it to go, you can take some charge of your body.

And now, I'm going to be quiet for a minute or two, and while I'm quiet, perhaps you'll want to continue to think about that golden light doing all the things you want it to do. I'm going to be quiet starting now.

[pause 60 seconds]

And now, with that golden light still within you . . . that powerful, vigorous, vital golden light still within you, that golden light that combines all of the power of the universe and of your body, and of any medication or radiation or any-thing else you're taking . . . with all of that still within you . . . and completely at your command . . . from now and forever . . . perhaps you'll see yourself stand up on the beach. And as you stand on the beach . . . if you want to . . . visualize yourself without any physical problem whatsoever, and see what feel-ing comes over you without any physical problem what-soever. And know that that's *your* feeling and that you can call on that feeling at any time. You can call on that feeling, or you can call on the golden light, or you can call on the feeling of security at any time without interfering in any way with all of the things that you're doing.

And now perhaps, if you'd like, see yourself at the bottom of the same flight of stairs you just came down, and we'll walk up those stairs together. When you reach the top of the stairs, you will be back at a place where you started, feeling completely alert, and at least as well as you felt when we started, and most likely much better . . . and take the first step up. And now the second step up [speak slowly here] . . . and the third, and the fourth, and the fifth . . . and you're halfway up . . . and when you reach the tenth step, you'll be back in the place where you started, feeling completely alert and at least as well as you felt when you started and, perhaps and most likely, much better.

And now you can open your eyes at any time. And now take the next step up, and you're back at the place where you started . . . feeling completely alert and at least as well as you felt when you started, and most likely much better . . . and you can open your eyes at any time.

---

34. Script for directed visualization for chemotherapy or radiation

❧

PROCEDURE FOR LISTENING TO DIRECTED VISUALIZATIONS

- **This exercise can be used before, during, and after your treatment.**
- **If it is used before or after the treatment, allot twenty minutes.**
- **Sit quietly where you can be alone and quiet for that period of time.**
- **Play the tape. It contains all the instructions.**
- **Make a conscious effort to follow directions.**

The script should be read slowly and deliberately into a

tape recorder in your normal voice. Pause periodically so that when you listen to the tape, you will have time to absorb the instructions.

This is going to be a time of complete relaxation...a conscious effort to relax as completely as possible and to do all you can so the chemotherapy (or radiation) will be as effective and as comfortable for you as possible. Get into as comfortable a position as you can, and close your eyes. For the next couple minutes, just concentrate on your breathing.

To the best of your ability, see your lungs...see how they feel, consciously see how they feel while they're completely expanded, and see how they feel after you exhale. Be aware that there's no right way and no wrong way to do what you're doing now...that whatever results you get are perfect results, and that if all you do is relax, that's wonderful. This is not a time to be worrying about any of the things that are happening in your day-to-day life. This is a time only for you, and you can let it all hang out. For this very short period of time, you can completely relax. You are never out of control. You can feel completely secure.

Now, once again, concentrate on your lungs. Picture them in your mind's eye. See if you can see them filled...see if you can see them after you relax. And if your mind drifts away, and you want to, just bring it slowly back to where you are or where you want it to be. You're doing nothing wrong, and anything you do will be a success. And if you hear my voice, that'll be fine...and if you don't, that's fine, too. You can be absolutely sure that your subconscious is hearing every word I say.

And now, perhaps, in your mind's eye—way, way out in space—you can see a word all lit up...and the word is RE-LAX. Just relax...and now that same word is about a foot in front of your forehead...just see it about a foot in front of your forehead, the word RELAX. And now inside your forehead, see that word, and just relax.

Now perhaps, if you want to, pay attention to your left

foot, and the toes on your left foot, and your ankle, and let them all relax . . . and all the cares and tensions of the day just drain down into the floor. Consciously let them relax . . . and any noise you hear will only serve to deepen your relaxation.

And now pay attention, if you will, to your right shoulder. All the muscles of your right shoulder, completely relaxed. All the cares of the day drain away and leave you. And consciously check your right shoulder to see if there's any tension there. Think about it. And now all of the muscles and tendons of your right foot, and the toes of your right foot, and the ankle, just let them relax. And now the calf of your right leg, let it relax. And for this very short period of time in your mind's eye, perhaps you can see that wonderfully long bone running from your ankle to your knee in your right leg . . . See how wonderfully straight and long and solid it is . . . and what a wonderful feat of construction. Let it relax . . . let all the muscles just relax . . . and the muscles of your left calf . . . relax. And way, way out in the future, there's that word RELAX . . . way, way into the future.

And now let all the muscles of your left shoulder completely relax . . . Let it just droop toward the ground . . . and rest comfortably against the seat you're in. Let it relax. And now the muscles of your stomach. Let your stomach just hang out . . . just relaxed. Once again, it's like when you were a very, very little person, just learning how to do all of the things you had to do, like telling time and reading . . . And now the muscles of your left thigh . . . This is a time for relaxation . . . and you don't have to go to sleep . . . but if you do, that's fine . . . and if my voice drifts away, that's fine . . . and if your mind drifts away, that's fine, too. Whatever you do is wonderful. Completely relax.

And now all the muscles of the right thigh . . . just let them relax. All the tensions of the day just drain out of them into the seat below you. And there's that word RELAX. Consciously in your mind is the word RELAX way, way out in the past . . . just in the past . . . and right behind your forehead.

And all the muscles of your face now . . . the muscles of

your lips, your cheeks, and your forehead, just let them fall toward the ground and your stomach. And your chest... once again, your chest just relaxed, and now your back, and your complete right arm and the fingers of your right hand. And if there's any part of your body that's not completely relaxed already, it soon will be.

You may be surprised to see how relaxed you are already. That may come as a surprise to you... and as I said, if there's any part of your body that's not yet relaxed, it soon will be. And if there's any part of your body that's not feeling as comfortable as it might, concentrate on that part of the body for the next few seconds... just think of it... and send all the endorphins of the brain down in that area. Consciously be aware of any part of your body that's not as comfortable as it might be.

And now all the muscles and sinews and tendons of your left arm and your left hand and the fingers of your left hand completely relax. And all the muscles of your neck and your shoulders and your chest and your buttocks and the whole pelvic area now... Think about the whole pelvic area... once again your face... and your head... And if my voice drifts away, that's fine, just as long as you're sitting back comfortably and relaxing.

Many things are changing in your body, all of which are normal and wonderful, just through your relaxation.

And now, perhaps, if you want to, you'll see yourself at the top of a flight of ten steps going down. You've been at the top of stairs before, and you will be again. So this is completely familiar to you. This is a time when you can just put your trust in the world. You will never be out of control in any way. You can trust... like you did when you were a very, very little person. And everything is going to turn out exactly as you want it to. We're going to walk down these steps together, if you want to, and with every step down you take, you're going to relax just a little bit more.

And now, if you will, you can take the first step down... and you've taken one step down, and you have nine to go. And with every step down, you relax just a little bit more. And any noise you hear will serve to relax you just a little bit more. And way, way out in the future, and way, way back in the past, and right behind your forehead is that word RELAX.

And now, you take another step down. And with every step down you relax just a little bit more, and now you've taken two steps down, and you have eight steps to go... And take another step down... relaxing just a little bit more with every step you go down. And feel that relaxation in your body... and you may be surprised at how relaxed you feel already. And now take another step down, and that's four steps down, and you have six to go. This is a time for relaxation. It's not necessary for you to go to sleep, but if you want to, that's fine. If it happens, that's fine; or if your mind drifts away, that's fine. Nothing that you do is wrong.

Take one more step down. And now you're halfway down the stairs... You have five more steps to go... And you take another step down. And see yourself, consciously see yourself, on the sixth step down, and how comfortable you feel, and how secure you feel, and how trusting you feel. And now another step down... and now you've taken seven steps down and you have three to go. And there's that word RELAX shining way, way out in the heavens and behind your forehead at the same time... and you take another step down... and you've taken eight steps and you have two more to go. And now one more step... and you've taken nine steps down and you have one to go... and now take that last step down, and you're all the way down to the bottom of the stairs. And you may be surprised at how relaxed you really are.

And now, visualize yourself in the circumstances you are in when you take the chemotherapy (or radiation)—the treatment that is going to destroy the cancer cells in your body—and see how relaxed you are, how comfortable you are, and how sure you are that the treatment is going to do exactly what you want it to do. And see the medicine as an elixir, a magic potion, a friend... as a golden light... that goes directly to the place or places in your body where the cancer cells—

those weak, erratic, confused little cells—are located. And they are hiding because the strong and powerful medicine you are taking—that golden light—will hunt them out, crush them, and destroy them. And it will do all that with the least amount of nausea or uncomfortable feelings. The golden light is so much more powerful than the cancer cells, yet is soothing and gentle to all other parts of your body. When the chemotherapy is being administered, you can call down all the endorphins from your brain to do whatever is necessary so that there is the least amount of discomfort.

Then squeeze your right fist, which is a sign that you are calling down all of the power of the universe to join with the medicine and your own mental and physical strengths to ensure that the medicine does everything it was designed to do...in the shortest amount of time and with the least amount of discomfort. Squeeze your right fist...squeeze it hard.

And now, if you feel like it and if you want to, visualize yourself as completely well...without any illness and without any discomfort. See how that feels...Think about it now. And then, when you are taking the chemotherapy (or radiation), remember this feeling and squeeze your right hand and hopefully, that feeling of calmness, relaxation, and comfort will return...And hopefully, that will serve to energize all the powers of your mind, all the powers of your body, all the powers of the medicine, and all the powers of the universe to join together to do exactly what the medicine is supposed to do—in the shortest possible time and with the least amount of discomfort...Take as long as you want right now to enjoy that feeling, so that you can remember it and regain it at such time as you need it...

And now, that golden light is still within you...that powerful, vigorous, vital golden light still within you...that golden light that combines all of the power of the universe and of your body...all of it completely at your command... from now and forever.

Now, see yourself at the bottom of the same flight of

stairs you just came down, and we'll walk up those stairs together. When you reach the top of the stairs, you will be back at a place where you started, feeling completely alert, and at least as well as you felt when we started, and most likely much better... and take the first step up. And now the second step up [speak slowly here]... and the third, and the fourth, and the fifth... and you're halfway up... and when you reach the tenth step, you'll be back in the place where we started, feeling completely alert, and at least as well as you felt when we first started, and most likely much better... and take the next step up, and now the seventh... and the eighth... and the ninth step... And when you take the next step, you'll be back in the place where you started... feeling completely alert and at least as well as you felt when you started and, perhaps and most likely, much better.

And now you can open your eyes at any time. And now take the next step up, and you're back at the place where you started... feeling completely alert and at least as well as you felt when you started, and most likely much better... and you can open your eyes at any time.

---

35. Can love play a part in the fight for recovery?

☙

Love is one of the most potent immune-system enhancers! Here is what we now know about it:

There is scientific evidence that negative emotions have a negative effect on the immune system, and that positive emotions enhance the immune system. We can extrapolate from that research that the more powerful the emotion, the more extreme its effect on the immune system. Since love is one of the most powerful of all the positive emotions, it is also among the most potent immune-system enhancers.

For those reasons, everyone would be well-served to direct his efforts to loving, or at least liking, as many of the persons, places, things, and events encountered in life as possible.

How can you increase loving feelings in your life? One way is to "act as if" you feel love; if you do this long enough and consistently enough (see chapter 30), love may actually emerge. Also, as you will see in chapter 38, joining with others to fight a common enemy or to seek a common cause—knowing that they depend on you and you depend on them—often arouses feelings of warmth and closeness. And revealing your foibles and idiosyncrasies to others and learning about theirs (as described in chapter 38) can be the basis for deep, lasting mutual affection.

Another way to turn negative emotions into more positive ones is to analyze your feelings of distaste for others. If you search for the answer as to why you don't like someone or something, you will often find that the reasons for your negative reaction are unimportant and relatively easy to overcome. If you're like me, it's much easier to learn *not to dislike* another person than it is to learn to love him.

So the next time you find yourself in a situation where you don't like someone or something, ask yourself why, and then ask whether the whole subject is worth the stress produced by that negative reaction. Since you will often find that your dislike is based on trivial matters, your reaction will often change from dislike to a neutral position. Although perhaps not as healthful as loving, this is still a major step toward the positive emotions that may enhance the power of the immune system—in addition to making us a good deal happier.

But as you try to love and rid yourself of negative reactions to the people and events around you, if your illness does not progress as you think it should, it's not because you're not loving well enough. No one can love more or better than you can. It's unrealistic to believe that if you love enough, your recovery is guaranteed. Loving is an emotion to be cherished and enjoyed, not an obligation or duty.

---

36. Can laughter assist my recovery process?

Laughter in and of itself cannot cure cancer nor prevent cancer, but laughter as part of the full range of positive emotions including hope, love, faith, strong will to live, determination and purpose, can be a significant and indispensable aspect of the total fight for recovery.

That statement is a compilation of many statements made by Norman Cousins over the last several years. In order to fully understand it, you need the following background information.

In 1979 Cousins—then the editor of *The Saturday Review* and now an adjunct professor at the UCLA School of Medicine and honorary chairman of The Wellness Community's Board of Trustees—published *Anatomy of an Illness*. In that book, Cousins described his fight with and recovery from a disease called ankylosing spondylitis, which he described as "a disintegration of the connective tissue of the spine—a particularly painful, debilitating, and sometimes fatal disease."

In the 172-page paperback edition of his book, Cousins devoted approximately one-and-one-half pages to his experiment with laughter. Here's what he wrote:

It was easy enough to hope, love, and have faith, but what about laughter? Nothing is less funny than being flat on your back with all the bones in your spine and joints hurting. A systematic program was indicated. A good place to begin, I thought, was with amusing movies. Allen Funt, producer to the spoofing television program "Candid Camera," sent films of some of his "CC" classics, along with a motion-picture projector. The nurse was instructed in its use. We were even able to get our hands on some old Marx Brothers films. We pulled down the blinds and turned on the machine.

It worked. I made the joyous discovery that ten minutes of genuine belly-laughter had an anesthetic effect and would give me at least two hours of pain-free sleep. When the pain-killing effects of the laughter wore off, we would switch on the motion-picture projector again, and not infrequently, it would lead to another pain-free sleep interval. Sometimes the nurse read to me out of a trove of humor books. Especially useful were E. B. and Katherine White's *Subtreasury of American Humor* and Max Eastman's *The Enjoyment of Laughter.*

How scientific was it to believe that laughter —as well as the positive emotions in general—was affecting my body chemistry for the better? If laughter did in fact have a salutary effect on the body's chemistry, it seemed at least theoretically likely that it would enhance the system's ability to fight the inflammation. (It seemed to be working.) I was greatly elated by the discovery that there is a physiologic basis for the ancient theory that laughter is good medicine.

Although the description of his laughter experiment was quite brief, many people interpreted the main message of the book to be that laughter had "cured" him. Cousins, in the *Los Angeles Times* in October 1985, called that interpretation of his statements an "absurd notion."

To the best of my knowledge, no one has ever argued that laughter can cure cancer or any other disease. However, as part of the total range of positive emotions, laughter may have a salutary effect on the recovery process.

Laughter and humor have always been an integral part of The Wellness Community program. At social events, and whenever members get together just to be with one another, merriment and joyfulness are abundant. Laughter, giggling, chortling, good will, banter, hugging, friendship, and love are essential parts of everything we do. It's not that we go out of our way to make them happen. It's just that they are a natural result of people being together to help each other.

When Allen Funt of "Candid Camera" came to the Community to film a segment for a TV show, he asked one participant, "Do you believe that laughter really does you any good —not because other people have told you that it should, but because you have experienced it?" The answer:

> I know laughter is good for me. I don't know if it is helping me get better, but it makes me feel better— not only mentally but physically as well—and it takes my mind off my own situation. Life and its pleasures have become very real to me and I know just how important it is to enjoy each enjoyable minute. So when something strikes me as laughable, I laugh. I want to be conscious of every joyful part of life.
>
> Before cancer, I only paid attention to the problems of life, the need and difficulty of making a living, maintaining relationships, and getting ahead. The frustrating and hurtful incidents were the ones I related to my friends when they said, "How are things?" Occasionally, we talked about the good times, but it seems to me that what I did the most of was complain, and I took the pleasant and joyful parts of life as routine and as my due.
>
> That's all different now. Now I accentuate the

positive and eliminate the negative.... Most importantly, I make sure that I am aware of the good times when they come along. So when something is funny, I laugh; and that reinforces my certainty that life is good.

Laughter may also be good for cancer for physical reasons. Laughter relieves stress, which may make it possible for the immune system to become stronger. Studies by William Fry, M.D., of Stanford University and Paul Ekman, Ph.D., of the University of California, San Francisco, tested the immune systems of participants before and after laughter or smiling, and both concluded that "laughter/humor resets the immune system."

In addition, the more laughter there is, the higher the quality of life; and the higher the quality of life, the greater the will to live.

At The Wellness Community, when we became aware of the possible benefits of laughter, we conducted a Joke Fest. Because the *Los Angeles Times* described so well the way Victors use laughter as part of their fight for recovery, excerpts are reprinted here from the article by journalist Dick Roraback. It carried the headline, "Cancer Is a Laughing Matter at This Clinic":

"Anybody have a good cancer joke?" the moderator asks. Half a dozen hands go up. "Great," he says. "Try to top this one...."

Bowdlerized version: A man stops by his doctor's office to get the result of a check-up. The doctor tells him he has cancer.

"How long do I have?"

"I'm sorry. Just until tonight."

The man goes home, tells his wife. When they finish crying, he suggests that they go upstairs and fool around, just one last time.

"Golly, Herb," she says, "I'd love to but I'm really too tired."

"Aw, come on," he urges, "just for old time's sake."

"Sure, that's easy for you to say," she replies. "You don't have to get up in the morning." ...

The conversation drifts back to endorphins and their possible effect on the immune system.

"They're secreted by the brain," somebody explains. "They supply a natural morphine-like substance for pain relief."

Another suggests that meditation can release endorphins; extended exercise as well. Still another asks Jeff, who brought up the subject in the first place, whether smiling is enough, or do you have to actually laugh out loud.

"I'm not sure," Jeff says, "but I do know that good sex releases good endorphins, too."

"Sure," a friend says, "especially if your partner is laughing at you." ...

"Science is finally catching up to what people have known intuitively forever," one man says, "that laughter is the best medicine. Chicken soup, too."

"At least for the time you're laughing," a woman says, "you're not even thinking about stress." ...

"It's important not to take things too seriously. Even your cancer. Don't even take life seriously. You'll never get out of it alive."

So *give yourself permission to laugh and enjoy life, and make sure that your family and friends permit you to laugh.* Most people without cancer believe that people with cancer are always sad and despairing, and whenever they come in contact with a cancer patient, they adopt a sad and sympathetic look. Under those circumstances, it's easy to act the part of the doomed object of pity and give up all laughter and fun. But don't do it—and don't let them do it to you.

Your friends don't mean to get in the way of your enjoyment of life. They just believe that the only way to act around a cancer patient is downcast, unhappy, and sympathetic. Straighten them out. Tell them you want them to act with you as they did before the illness. Point out that you want to enjoy life.

As one woman at the Joke Fest said, "I found that laughter isn't just fun, it's essential." As oncologist Michael B. Van Scoy-Mosher has commented, one characteristic of the cancer patient who does well is the ability to often "put cancer in the background for periods of time" (see chapter 27). Laughter and being involved with other peoples' lives—as well as going on with love, fun, and involvement in your own life—is one way to do this. The statement "It's fun to laugh" may be redundant, but it's meaningful.

---

37. Would being around other cancer patients really be beneficial for me?

There are two basic reasons why cancer patients don't want to be with others who have the same disease. First, many of them want to forget they have cancer, and the presence of others with the illness is a constant reminder. Second, they don't want to feel the sadness and fear that would be engendered by the death or physical deterioration of a newfound friend. Many patients ask, "Why should I go out of my way to become friends with or even become acquainted with someone who may die soon?"

Many Wellness Community participants have overriden such feelings in the quest for recovery. They believe, in fact, that their newfound relationships with other cancer patients have been the major benefit of the The Wellness Community program. They say that being with other cancer patients can foster a certain calmness that is difficult if not impossible to achieve around well persons. Lack of understanding is a major impediment to a relationship between cancer patients and those who do not have cancer. It is impossible for any well person to appreciate the always-nagging fear and the lack of control that impinge upon every area of life, and how the illness makes it difficult to make even the simplest plans.

These same people tell me that "we cancer patients, on the other hand, share an enormous number of experiences unknown to all but the initiated." They know how uncomfortable it is to automatically evoke pity from someone you meet for the first time, solely because of the illness. They have shared the feelings in the pit of the stomach when the diagnosis was first made, and the anxieties that keep them awake in the middle of the night. They understand the apprehension about the future and the despondency caused by chemotherapy and its side effects. And they have learned that life goes on after the diagnosis and that there is always room for hope.

This matter was addressed at a Sharing Group by Greg, a 26-year-old cancer patient. Greg has since moved from Los Angeles and I have lost track of him. But when last seen, he had been told that he was completely without symptoms. As a Victor, he told others:

> Other cancer patients have gone through what you are going through, so they can relate to you. They don't give you pity. But your parents and friends—however much they love you—can't relate to your struggle. They offer you sympathy without understanding, which is better than nothing, but people, particularly people with cancer, need to be understood.

Another participant, who has been without symptoms of

cancer for over a year, also provided great insight into the reasons why being with other cancer patients is less stress-producing than being with well people:

> Up until recently I, too, always felt a great deal of strain being with most of my well friends. The reasons for that stress now appear very obvious to me. I found myself constantly shielding them from my real fears and pain so that they wouldn't be devastated. Or I was fighting back my annoyance because they didn't really comprehend the seriousness of the matter, or I was irked by the fact that they were not relating to me in the same way they did before. And sometimes I was resentful and jealous because they were well and I was ill, and at other times I thought they felt superior to me for the same reason. With other cancer patients, on the other hand, I relaxed. Those emotions weren't appropriate.

Some cancer patients describe the benefit they receive from being with other cancer patients in terms of an esprit de corps. They recognize that they are experiencing the same warmth of togetherness so prevalent in groups of people who have joined together to fight a common enemy—people such as soldiers, firefighters, and police officers.

The basic emotion expressed by many cancer patients could be summed up in this statement: "I want to be with you because you understand, because you see in me what I see in you, because your well-being is important to me, and I know that you want the best for me and care what happens to me. I don't have to explain to you, nor do I need to hide from you, either the fears or the hopes for the future that lie deep inside me, because you are feeling those same fears and hopes."

Actress Jill Ireland Bronson commented on The Wellness Community in a recent magazine article:

> When you have cancer, you feel very isolated. It's

important to be with other people who have cancer. You feel normal, not singled out. You don't feel
that you're odd or a freak. And people don't look at
you with a great fear in their eyes. You might even
find that there are others in worse condition than
you, and you can help them. That's a good feeling.

At a recent meeting, one participant drew an interesting
analogy. He proposed that there was a great similarity between cancer patients and people who are part of a common
disaster, such as a flood or a hurricane. He based his analogy
on an article he had read that indicated that people who
joined together to help each other in times of crisis experience a feeling of togetherness very few had ever experienced
before.

The article he mentioned was a study by UCLA researcher Linda Nelson, Ph.D. After studying people involved in
more than twenty natural disasters over the past sixty years,
Dr. Nelson concluded, "Residents in the stricken communities
generally keep their heads, care for one another, share common resources, and *actually reach an emotional high as
they pull together and tackle the common challenges of
survival and rebuilding.* Many of them," she added, "feel
saddened at some level when the crisis is over; they realize
that they have never experienced that emotion before and
perhaps never will again."

In the same way, the cancer patient faces an enormous
challenge and, while pulling together with others to beat the
odds, can reach an emotional high. And perhaps so will you.

Several studies have proved that cancer patients benefit
from being with other cancer patients. One such study, published in 1983 by the Rand Corporation, was titled "Measuring
the Ability to Cope with Serious Illness." Its author, Anita
Stewart, Ph.D., wrote, "It has been suggested that seriously ill
people have a particular need for support from other seriously ill patients—i.e., from others who have experienced

the same problems and feelings." And she pointed out "that people cope more effectively with disability when they have a firm sense of belonging in a highly valued group such as a family or community."

A large number of cancer telephone hot lines, the function of which is to match up cancer patients with others, are springing up around the country. This is another indication that cancer patients need and want to be with one another.

The primary reason for seeking out other cancer patients is to improve the quality of your life in the hope or belief that this will enhance the possibility of your recovery. However, no one is suggesting that you spend all of your time with other cancer patients. That would be just as counterproductive as spending no time with them. But as I indicated at the beginning of this section, most of the participants at The Wellness Community believe that their relationships with other cancer patients have been *the* major benefit of the program. You may find the same to be true for you.

There is one more issue to be addressed here: the reluctance of some cancer patients to become friends with others with cancer for fear that the emotional trauma would be devastating if the newfound friend does not do as well as hoped. Although this is a legitimate cause for misgivings, the relevant question here is, "Shall I forgo the possible benefits and pleasures of a new friend who has cancer—and who therefore understands me better than anyone else can—because of the *possibility* that the relationship will end sooner than I want it to?"

All our participants have opted in favor of friendship. They have integrated into their psyche the concept that one has no alternative but to accept the eventuality of the death of a friend as a part of life, and that it is in their best interests to appreciate the joy of the present with full knowledge of the tenuousness of the future.

In conversations among participants after the death of one of our friends, there is certainly a sense of loss. But the

dominant theme is always how lucky we were to have enjoyed the benefits of the relationship, and how sorry we
would have been to have missed them.

If you want to give it a try, you can find other cancer
patients wherever you are. Ask your doctor, or call the American Cancer Society in your area. Look up a hot line in your
area in the Yellow Pages under "Cancer." In all but the most
remote regions of the country, there are organizations that
will help you find other cancer patients. Most of The Wellness
Community participants would recommend that you take the
chance. And they would assure you that the odds are very
good that you will experience the same benefit out of being
with other cancer patients as they did. Go for it! Good luck!

38. What is a support group and how can it help me?

೪

Group therapy as an effective tool in the Patient Active's fight
for recovery is not a new concept. Chronically ill people
participated in such groups as early as the turn of the cen-
tury, and their popularity burgeoned in the 1970s. In her
1980 American Psychological Association Presidential address, Leona Tyler, M.D., who has done extensive research in
this field, suggested that by the year 2000, support groups
will be the primary vehicle for dealing with health-related
psychosocial issues.

How important can these groups be? In Jane Goldberg's
book, *Psychotherapeutic Treatment of Cancer Patients,* N.
Miller, M.D., an authority on the subject, is quoted thus: "Lim-
iting the treatment [of cancer] to medical remedies only is

analogous to trying to save a sinking ship by bailing out the water while ignoring the holes in the bottom of the ship."

At a 1976 American Cancer Society conference on group counseling with cancer patients and their families, Irving Yalom, M.D., of the Stanford Medical School ended his address by saying:

> Some of the [cancer] patients who have worked most effectively in a group have come very far. What we've seen is that the confrontation [with a life-threatening illness in the group] for many people has resulted in a richer mode of living... than was true for them before their cancer. They are able to trivialize the trivia in their lives and alter their life perspective—not to do things they really don't want to do.... It's kind of a liberating feeling involving more willingness to take risks... and perhaps setting certain goals.

I suggest that you seriously consider seeking this type of support as part of your fight for recovery for two reasons: To become part of an intimate and closely knit group of people; and to reduce stress.

The most important of these reasons is the former—to gain an extended family who will make unwanted aloneness impossible. I'm defining "extended family" as a number of people (one other person is better than none) who will discuss all aspects of any subject, including cancer; who treat you as a friend with cancer rather than as a doomed object of pity; who are not so threatened by the possible eventual outcome of the illness (as are most family members) that all conversations are stilted and awkward; who do not react to your day-to-day problems with resentment; and to whom your discomfort is not so devastating as to make social intercourse impossible.

The significance of this extended family cannot be overemphasized. As you've read in chapter 25, unwanted aloneness—along with feelings of hopelessness, helplessness, and loss of control—is one of the most crippling psychosocial impediments to the cancer patient's recovery. And one of the ideal means of warding off the ill effects of unwanted aloneness is a support group.

Kari, a free-lance writer in her mid-40s, attests to the importance of an extended family for cancer patients. Kari had had an adenocarcinoma surgically removed from her left lung about six months earlier:

> I became part of a group because I was terrified, and I didn't want to be alone. I wanted to be with people who were experiencing the same after-effects of cancer I was. I knew that something had invaded my body and had changed my life both physically and mentally forever, and I felt, and I still feel, a very strong need to be around people to whom I can talk, so that I don't feel alone. And when I'm scared, I know that there is someone who will listen to me and not be frightened by what I'm saying.
>
> If my mother asks me how I am, the question is so loaded with emotional overtones that a straight answer is almost impossible. If my friend becomes angry with me, she's afraid to show it—she's afraid of me since I became ill. But in my group, everybody is in the same boat and has experienced the same problems I have. I don't frighten them.
>
> From the group, we all receive the courage to keep trying. When you feel sick and vulnerable, it's very hard to keep going, to try to change things and take control. Without a group, I don't know how people "get it together" to say "I want this treatment" when Dr. A says one thing and Dr. B another, and your instincts tell you a third.
>
> One of the most important results of my participation in the group is that the group became the

catalyst for learning the lessons cancer had to teach. If I'm depressed about something unrelated to cancer, I can bring it to my group. And by hearing how others would handle the same situation, I learn new methods of attacking problems, and I can get rid of the stress in my life.

I have also learned many skills in my group that I can use the rest of my life. For instance, I have learned to talk to myself. When I face a problem, I consciously discuss the various possibilities with myself and with others. That helps a lot in making the right decision.

Not only is it healthy to have many social contacts, but there is no question that the deeper, the more meaningful, and the longer-lasting the friendships are, the healthier they are. And there is no better way to build such relationships than to be with other people in a support group in which you expose your weaknesses and foibles and ask for help, and in which others do the same with you.

Another reason for becoming involved in a support group is to reduce the stress in your life. Here are the facts and theories (all of which we have discussed before) that lead to that conclusion. Taken together, they make the reasons for being in a support group that much more compelling:

1. We all have cancer cells growing in our bodies at all times. (Fact)

2. If unchecked, those cancer cells can multiply and grow into tumors and become one of more than 100 diseases known as cancer. (Fact)

3. Under normal circumstances, our immune systems seek out and destroy the cancer cells before they can get a foothold. (Fact)

4. Stress depresses the power of the immune system. (Fact)

5. Perhaps stress weakened your immune system sufficiently to permit the cancer to take hold in your body.
(Theory)

6. Perhaps the stress in your life, at this time exacerbated by the trials of the disease, continues to depress
the immune system, thereby making recovery more
difficult. (Theory)

7. Perhaps if the stress is eliminated or ameliorated,
the immune system will become stronger and alter
the course of the disease toward health. (Theory)

8. Many professionals believe that being in a group is
the most effective way of reducing stress.

Wellness Community groups include only cancer patients
over twenty-one, and participants can remain in them as long
as they consider necessary. They are led by licensed psycho-
therapists and are not "rap" groups.

We do not permit our groups to meet in either a place of
religious worship or a medical establishment. The reason for
these restrictions is that our program is concerned only with
the psychological, social, and philosophical, and we hope that
our participants "solve" their psychological "problems" themselves, using our staff for advice and observations. If the meetings were held in a medical establishment, individuals would
likely turn to an authority—a physician—for answers when
they come to a difficult place in the road. If meetings were
held in a place of religious worship, they might turn to an
even higher authority.

As I describe our groups, I am fully aware that The Wellness Community is one of the few places where this type of
group is available. Because of that, in order to be in a group,
you should be willing to compromise. If the group you find
doesn't have other cancer patients, is time-limited, is in a
church or a hospital, or is segregated by disease or age, *use it.*
If you can't find any group at all, *start one* (see chapter 39).
However, avoid any group that seems to believe that cancer

patients are doomed and wants only to make you comfortable with that prospect.

You might consider private therapy if you can afford it, or look for a facility where you can receive counseling without charge. Be sure that the therapist understands what you are looking for and knows that you are in therapy because you believe or hope it will help your recovery process. While private therapy can't give you the social contacts or the extended family you need, it can help you find areas of stress in your life.

However, if the therapist wants to teach you to take a resigned, passive stance vis-à-vis your diagnosis and prognosis—and that's all he or she wants to do—that therapist is not for you. You want to be a Patient Active. You want to fight for your recovery.

By reaching out to others, you can experience what one of our participants described this way:

> My group is part of my family. But what I really learned from my fellow cancer patients is that I can also share enough of me with my friends and be interested enough in them so that they become like family, too. Now my family just keeps growing and my group becomes my family and my family becomes my group. It all works.

To find a support group, call the American Cancer Society; or write Make Today Count, P.O. Box 222, Sage Beach, Maryland 65065; or We Can Do, 129 North Mayflower, Monrovia, California 91016. You can also contact the Self-Help Resource Center, 2349 Franz Hall, Psychology Department, 405 Hilgard Avenue, UCLA, Los Angeles, California 90024; telephone 800-222-5465.

39. How do I form a support group if I can't find one?

If you want to start a support group, you don't have to go to great lengths. Find two or three other cancer patients who are of a like mind and arrange to meet with them. If you do nothing more than compare notes and experiences, it will be worthwhile. And in the ensuing weeks, it's quite possible that more cancer patients will learn of your group and want to join.

As you get your group off the ground, keep these general parameters in mind, while acknowledging that they can be modified to suit your needs and circumstances:

- The group should consist of between three and twelve people who meet on a regular basis (probably once a week) to discuss matters of mutual concern, with the understanding that the group is another method of fighting for recovery, along with chemotherapy or other medical treatment.

- Ideally, all of the members should be cancer patients.

- In order to build an "extended family" and reduce stress, get to know the people in the group as well as possible.

- The group should not spend an appreciable amount of time discussing religious, medical, or nutritional matters; the focus should be kept on learning as much about each other as possible.

- Everyone must understand that the cancer patients are not using the group to learn only to cope with the illness or to make the best of things while waiting for the disease to take its toll.

• For reasons set out in chapter 38, avoid having the group meet in a medical/hospital setting or a place devoted to religious activities. ˜

• If possible, the group should be led by a licensed psychotherapist.

• Each session should probably last between ninety minutes and two hours.

For help in starting your self-help group, contact the Self-Help Resource Center, 2349 Franz Hall, Psychology Department, 405 Hilgard Avenue, UCLA, Los Angeles, California 90024 (phone 800-222-5465).

To locate other cancer patients, ask your doctor for some names or call a cancer hot line. The National Coalition for Cancer Survivorship (323 8th Street, Albuquerque, New Mexico 87102; phone 505-764-9956) will probably be able to help you find a hot line in your community. So can the American Cancer Society.

Finally, if you can't find a group or start one, ask a friend to help you use as many as possible of the concepts set out here and in chapter 40. Allowing other people to get to know the real you can be a worthwhile and health-enhancing experience.

40. How can I get the most out of a support group?

❧

Once you become part of a group, or decide to be open with a friend or friends, treat the experience as an important part of your total care. Get down to essentials as soon as possible—that is, talk about yourself. Reveal as much about yourself as you can. Tell the others in your group about matters you have never discussed before.

You probably will fib and shade the truth in the beginning. Everybody does. But be as honest and open as you can. You are doing it *for you*. The faster you find out what parts of your life you are hiding—which are therefore stress-producing—the sooner you can do something about them. And the more quickly you become true friends with your group-mates, the sooner you will reap the benefits of those friendships.

We expend an enormous amount of time and energy hiding facts about our feelings, beliefs, and things we have done. That energy could be spent instead on many more worthwhile efforts, such as fighting to get well.

Patients Active don't suggest that you tell every secret about yourself; obviously, there are some things it makes good sense to keep private. But they do suggest that you *know* what your secrets are, and decide whether it's worth the energy to keep them.

One way to discover the secrets in your life is to make a list of them. Start by asking yourself:

- What don't you want your friends to know about things you have done?
- About what you fantasize?
- About what you want out of life?

- About what is wrong with you physically or mentally?

- About what you're afraid of?

- About what ways you feel inadequate?

- What is there about you that you think would make your friends like you less if they knew it?

It may take a lot of thought to make your list, because most of us keep secrets even from ourselves. But stick to it. You have nothing to lose, and you may gain a lot.

Don't worry about the ramifications of writing these thoughts and memories on paper; you can burn it as soon as you're through. But such a list of secrets can be helpful, whether or not you join a support group.

One of the immediate benefits of the list is that after you make it, you will know that you have secrets and what they are. Before that, you probably weren't even aware that there were so many areas of your life that you couldn't or wouldn't talk about. Even if you did know of your secretiveness, it was probably so amorphous and ill-defined that there was no way to determine whether it was appropriate. The list also defines and separates the secrets so that you can look at each one and decide whether you ought to keep it secret. That way, you won't have to consider them all at once, which is impossible to do.

Constantly hiding something about yourself is a stressor, and the more secrets you keep, the more powerful those stressors are. So the best advice is, don't keep any more secrets than you have to.

If you are keeping a secret, consciously or unconsciously, it must be because you are somehow afraid that if someone else learns it, something unpleasant will happen. Perhaps they won't like or respect you as much, or you will get in trouble.

To determine whether your reasons for keeping secrets are rational, consider each one on your list and ask yourself why you can't discuss it with your friends. Will they like or respect you less? Be realistic. If the tables were turned and they revealed such a secret to you, how would you react? If your reason for keeping the secret turns out to be reasonable, then keep it. But if not, don't.

One Patient Active, a university professor, had the following experience:

> In the beginning, all of my secrets were very secret. I have always been a very private person. But soon I saw that not much was happening for me in the group, while some of the others who told a lot more about themselves seemed to be having a lot more fun. So I took a chance. I told them that I had failed several courses in high school. That had always been something I hid. I don't think I even knew I was hiding it. I guess I believed that if "they" knew about my failure, "they" wouldn't think I was as smart as I wanted "them" to.
>
> When I revealed that secret, and told them that even my wife didn't know about it, we all had a good laugh. With that experience under my belt, I became bolder and bolder, and it became easier and easier to tell more about myself. The funny thing is that the more they knew about me, the more they seemed to like me, and the better I felt about myself. People don't like or dislike you because of what you tell them. They make that decision based on how you treat them.

Some interesting things happen in the group setting. When you tell your group-mates or your friends about a specific situation in your life, you will find you are also telling them why you behaved the way you did. This can help you take a realistic look at your motivations and actions and decide whether they're working to your best advantage. If they're not, decide how you can improve the situation.

Furthermore, as you tell your group as much about yourself as you can, you'll probably find that they'll understand because they have had similar experiences. They will admire the fact that you took a risk and led the way. Most importantly, you will become their friend because you trusted them enough to tell them your secret and had confidence they would understand. You have made them special people in your life. And you will become a special person in their lives.

One caution: Some people talk with great animation when they are the subject of the conversation, but they sit back with a glazed look in their eyes when someone else is the center of attention. That doesn't work. People don't like people who are interested only in themselves. Dale Carnegie and every other writer who has ever offered advice about "winning friends and influencing people" have made it clear that to be liked, the first thing you must do is to make people believe you are interested in them. It works even better if you are *really* interested in their lives as well as your own.

If that's not your style, maybe it would be a good idea to try to change. It's easy: if you "act as if" you're interested in others for a while, you'll find that sooner or later you really will be. Try it.

Another reason to become interested in others is that it will take your mind off yourself. When you concentrate on someone else, you are putting your cancer in the background. You are taking the pressure of stress off your immune system for a while.

If your group-mates are not cancer patients, explain to them, as best you can, what being a cancer patient is like. Explain that, despite the myth that the diagnosis is a death sentence, cancer patients *can* fight for their lives, and that's exactly what you're doing. Tell them that cancer is not a curse or a punishment, but a disease like any other, and is nothing to be ashamed of; that many, many people with cancer recover and that you want to be one of them; that the more they know about you, the less need you will feel to hide who you are—and that that's good for your immune system. Enlist them in your fight for recovery. Let them know how important it is for you to have social contacts, to have people you can tell your fears to, without scaring them away.

As we know, they can never fully understand what it's like to have cancer. But they can try, and that will be good for both you and them. You might just be letting them in on a secret most people don't learn unless they become seriously ill: how important each day can be.

To sum up, you can get the most out of your group by telling as much as you can about yourself, by keeping as few secrets as possible, and by being interested in your group-mates. But don't expect instantaneous results. That's not the way it works. Hang in there; remember why you're there. You are a Patient Active, and you are fighting for your recovery. And if any of your group-mates are cancer patients, you will be fighting a common enemy and building an esprit that's not easily matched.

---

41. Why should I talk about my activities as a Patient Active?

❧

Telling your friends and others you meet about what you are doing to fight for your recovery can be an important part of that fight. Although I do not have any statistics to cite in support of this view, I have observed that those who get the best results from their efforts seem to talk about those efforts a lot.

The more you talk about the methods you are using to get well, the more you will understand and believe in those methods. In turn, the better you understand them, the more effective they will be. And when you answer the questions of others, you become a teacher instead of a student. To be a teacher requires that you convert what may be a rather vague notion into understandable language; and if you're like most of us, the one who will gain the most from that process is you.

One of our participants who had breast cancer with many complications over a seven-year period has now been without symptoms for almost two years. She often speaks about her activities as a Patient Active to various organizations. She looks forward to these speaking engagements she says, because:

> The one who learns the most from them is me.
>
> Every time I describe a technique I used, I learn another reason why it was so helpful and why I should continue to use it now.
>
> Because I have described so often the benefits of choosing between alternatives rather than reacting reflexively based on old memories, that method of taking control of my life has become second nature to me and is an important part of my happiness now. I'm not sure that I would have learned that lesson so quickly if I had not talked about it so much. Every time someone asks me a specific question about the Patient Active procedure, I'm forced to think more and more deeply and become more and more knowledgeable about the subject.

Don't underestimate the benefits to be gained by bragging about your efforts and the results you have achieved. While you are converting others to the belief that we all have some ability to control our own well-being, you will be reinforcing your own conviction. On the other hand, understand that the future is not all in your hands, and that the control you have over any situation is rather limited. The fact that you have chosen to take *any* control gives you a real edge.

42. Why should I continue chemotherapy or radiation when the side effects are so unpleasant?

❧

At the 1987 American Cancer Society conference, "Human Values and Cancer," James J. Strain, M.D., professor and director of consultation at Mount Sinai School of Medicine, spoke about patients' compliance with their physicians' instructions:

> Noncompliance with cancer chemotherapy undermines the successful application of proven therapies.... It has been shown by many studies that half or more of the patients observed failed to comply with the prescribed medical regimen. Clearly, noncompliance has a malignant effect upon survival.

It is not unusual for cancer patients to discontinue chemotherapy treatments, usually because they find the side effects so unpleasant and doubt whether the procedure will do any good. However, chemotherapy does seem to work in many cases. Gregory A. Curtis, M.D., deputy director of the National Cancer Institute's division of cancer treatment, wrote in a 1987 letter to the editor in the *Los Angeles Times:*

> During the 1950s, surgery and radiotherapy cured approximately 30 percent of cancer patients. Over the past thirty years, the improvements in radiotherapy *and the important discovery that drugs (chemotherapy) could actually cure advanced cancer have improved the curability rate to 50 percent*...Only 10 percent of the patients with the most aggressive of the lymphomas were expected

to survive five years in 1973. Today, 65 percent of these patients are curable. [Emphasis added.]

Giving up on chemotherapy is a decision to be made with great care. Unconscious noncompliance is not in your best interests.

---

43. Is it ever too late to begin the fight for recovery?

இ

In his book *The Body Is the Hero,* Ronald Glasser, M.D., tells a dramatic story that illustrates why it's never too late to try to alter the course of your illness.

A kidney containing unobserved cancer cells was transplanted into a recipient who had received drugs to suppress his immune system. (Unless the immune system is suppressed by drugs, it will reject a transplanted organ.)

Within days, the patient showed signs of cancer not only in his new kidney but also in his lungs. His doctors immediately deduced that the cancer had been introduced into his body by the transplanted kidney and had spread rapidly because his immune system had been rendered impotent by drugs. They discontinued the drugs. The cancer disappeared.

This story is a remarkable illustration of the power of the immune system. Weakened sufficiently to permit cancer cells to grow and take hold, it was able, when it regained its strength, to kill the cancer cells that had already started to form a tumor.

As shown in this case, a depressed immune system can regain enough strength to destroy a cancer that has already started to grow. Therefore, it's reasonable for you to hope that your immune system can be bolstered to reverse the course of the illness.

Every story of a recovered cancer patient teaches that same lesson.

IV
INTIMACY

44. How can I continue to enjoy intimacy and affection after cancer?

☙

The need and desire for sex, intimacy, and affection is a major area of concern for cancer patients and their partners. For most people, this subject is difficult to deal with even under the best of circumstances; with cancer in the picture, any feelings of sexual inadequacy, awkwardness, or insecurity that existed prior to the diagnosis become greatly magnified—at a time when the need to maintain the best possible relationships, particularly with sexual partners, is more important than ever. At the same time, the illness itself introduces new and difficult problems.

Obviously, cancer affects both sides of a sexually intimate relationship. If you're the cancer patient, your need for touching, holding, and loving may have increased, while your need for sexual intercourse may have decreased. If you're the partner or mate of a cancer patient, your need for sex and closeness continues as before, but it may have to be denied for some period of time.

Both partners, then, may be frustrated by changes, temporary or permanent, arising from the illness or the side effects of treatment. Intercourse may be out of the question because it's downright painful, impossible because of physical changes, or medically inadvisable. But, in all but the most extreme circumstances, the couple can solve most of these problems by enlarging their former range of intimate activities together.

The problems, of course, are psychological as well as physical. I have often heard the cancer patient say that he doesn't want to broach the subject with his partner because he's afraid she won't want to fondle or sleep with someone who has cancer or someone so mutilated. At the same time,

the well partner may be reluctant to make any advances toward intimacy, out of concern that the cancer patient's libido
is diminished since most of his energy is spent fighting the
illness. Who will speak first? What will happen if neither
speaks?

In this chapter, we will discuss the sexual and intimacy
problems brought about by cancer, and the ways many participants have resolved them. We will also look at some of the
findings of an extraordinarily thorough study called *Sexual
Side Effects of Cancer,* written by Marion E. Morra, assistant
director of the Yale Comprehensive Cancer Center, and her
colleagues and published by the National Cancer Institute.
Their conclusions are in line with the recommendations of
Wellness Community participants.

There are several basic premises agreed on in the study.
The first: "Each of us, no matter how young or old, healthy or
ill, regardless of marital status or sexual preference, has a
need to be loved and cared for and to share that love; these
needs continue even after the diagnosis; and one of the meaningful ways to meet such needs is sexual intimacy." Another
basic premise is that sex encompasses many different ways of
giving and receiving pleasure, even when intercourse is medically inadvisable, uncomfortable, or not desired.

Finally, everyone also agrees that communication is the
one indispensable element in the resolution of any sexual
problem. Solving a problem between two people is impossible
as long as the problem remains undefined and unenunciated.
Problems, particularly sexual problems, do not just go away if
ignored. Whether you are the cancer patient or the partner,
you must ask the questions you have on your mind. The
imagined answers to unasked questions keep most of us on
edge nearly all the time; for cancer patients, such uncertainty
is even more serious.

Ask for what you want. Dare to be the partner who
communicates clearly about what you would like, physically
as well as emotionally. If you learn only this lesson from this
chapter, it will be enough. Everything else will fall into place.

This advice is not always easy to follow, but if you decide not to start the conversation because you fear the worst, then you'd better resign yourself to fantasy, because fantasy is all you're going to get.

Most cancer patients experience some loss of sexual desire when cancer is a new element in their lives, or when treatment is at its worst. This lack of desire causes them much anxiety, magnified by the fear that it may be permanent. Usually, however, libido reappears as the stress or treatment decreases. Its return can be accelerated by love, tenderness, and openness between the partners.

As *Sexual Side Effects of Cancer* states:

> If the loss of interest in sex is caused by your feelings brought on by having cancer, it will probably be temporary and decrease as time goes on. If it is caused by medication, it will probably disappear when you go off the medication. If there is some physical cause, you and your partner should discuss that with your physician. It depends on the cause.

Keep in mind that sex doesn't necessarily mean sexual intercourse. The Yale report continues:

> Sex can mean a loving touch which has a special warmth that conveys feelings in a very direct way. Sitting or lying together, holding each other, cuddling, a warm hug, a hand squeeze, a kiss on the cheek, gentle stroking of the hair or a relaxing back rub are all ways of being sexual and fulfilling the need to be physically close.

Cancer or its treatment may affect your sexuality by dulling, eliminating, or slowing your response to touch. Changes in any part of the body often require major mental as well as physical adjustments. Reduced stamina and fatigue cause problems in intimacy as well as in other areas of life. Anger at

the illness sometimes gets directed toward one's sexual partner. Pain overwhelms sexuality. Depression reduces libido.

There is one particularly aggravating problem that is not
usually discussed, because of its convoluted nature. It will
become somewhat clearer, however, when seen through the
eyes of Oliver, a 48-year-old Wellness Community participant
with lymphoma:

> For weeks after I heard the diagnosis, I was so en-
> grossed in the emotions brought about by the ill-
> ness that the desire for closeness or sex was gone. I
> couldn't give my energy to anything but my recov-
> ery. I wanted Phyllis, my wife, to be loving and
> attentive but completely undemanding.
>
> But after a while, my conscience caught up
> with me. Phyllis was a young woman. Although she
> made no overtures, I was certain she was feeling
> the loss of sexuality as well as most other things in
> her life. I felt obligated to be affectionate—but it
> was hard work and not very pleasurable because I
> was so involved with myself.

Phyllis complained that Oliver had changed sexually and
that "sleeping with him as he is now is a chore." Both partners were "performing" out of feelings of duty, not love or
affection. And it wasn't working.

At the urging of their groups, Oliver and Phyllis started
to talk, and they soon arrived at solutions satisfactory to both.
These included specific changes in their lovemaking, as well
as a deeper understanding of how much they were willing to
do for each other. These discussions continue as they adjust
their intimate activities to the waxing and waning of the illness and their own emotional maturation process.

The lesson to be learned from Oliver and Phyllis is that
cancer can bring about feelings of selfishness and self-involve-
ment that shut out almost all emotions except the desire for a

solution, a cure, a reprieve. And one of the first emotions to go is the need to give pleasure—a topic that must be discussed and explored between you and your partner. If you do not feel sexual but you engage in sexual activity because you believe that's what your partner wants, that's OK—as long as you understand what you're doing and *don't resent it.* But if you do resent it, that feeling will fester and taint the relationship, perhaps forever.

There are times when the cancer patient is just not up to even thinking about sex or intimacy or a partner's needs. If and when that time comes, the only concern of either party should be the patient's comfort. There is no obligation to be involved in intimacy if you're not well enough. If sex is an obligation, it is not lovemaking, but only sex.

Now let's deal with some of the specifics related to sexuality and cancer, with the understanding that all the observations made here presuppose that both parties are interested in pursuing some type of sexual activity and it is not perceived as an obligation.

THE PAIN PROBLEM

Even if you are in pain most of the time, sex is not necessarily out of the question. If there are periods in the day or in the cycle of treatments when you feel better, you can plan intimacy for those times...and have something to fantasize about and look forward to.

A good time for shared intimacy may be after taking pain medication or after meditation and relaxation exercises. If you are still too uncomfortable for intercourse at these times, you may be able to participate in gentler types of sexual activity, like massage or stimulating sexual organs with oils or lotions.

If a scar is tender, try placing a pillow near the site of the incision or beneath it. Experiment with different positions until you come up with ones that put the least amount of weight or pressure on you. "Spoons" is one such position, where the couple lie side-by-side like spoons cradled one in the other.

The best method for making accommodations and new discoveries is to visualize, fantasize, and discuss them with your partner. Then try them.

THE FATIGUE FACTOR

As you probably know first-hand, feeling tired most of the time is not uncommon for cancer patients. And fatigue inhibits sexuality. Our participants often deal with this problem as they do with pain—by involving themselves in some less energetic activity, such as hugging, caressing, taking a shower together, or rubbing each other with oils.

However, while such foreplay might be good for the cancer patient, it may not satisfy the partner who isn't too tired to be aroused. In those circumstances, if the cancer patient desires the intimacy, he or she might consider satisfying the partner in some way that is not too physically demanding. This kind of intimacy can be planned for times when the cancer patient has just rested, meditated, or had a full night's sleep. Above all, sexual activity should not be planned after a heavy meal or consumption of alcohol.

THE BODY IMAGE ADJUSTMENT

Adjusting to a body change is sometimes the most difficult aspect of the illness. It takes time, effort, and thought to accept and integrate this new and unchangeable part of your life. But if you don't spend this time and effort, your new condition may relegate you to feeling unlovable and untouchable, perhaps forever.

The key here is to acknowledge your feelings of loss, shame, or embarrassment about the disfigurement of your body. With trusted loved ones, especially with your sexual partner, talk about those feelings, don't ignore them.

After an operation, many cancer patients hide the scar from their partner. But if the relationship is ever to be intimate and comfortable, such hiding cannot go on forever. Since it is inevitable that your partner see the scar sooner or later, make sure that you pick the time and place for the unveiling. Whether you do it with humor, solemnity, or something in between is up to you. However, be aware that your attitude can be the most significant factor in your partner's accommodation. If you see the bodily change as a romance-ending catastrophe, your partner may have difficulty seeing it as anything else.

None of this is easy. No one can tell you what will work for you. But one universal truth seems to emerge—namely, that there is the best chance of a happy ending when the two people involved tell each other the truth in a loving and caring way. So it's important that you accept what you cannot change, that your gratitude for what you have outweighs your sorrow for what you have lost, and that your delight in being alive shines through for all to see.

Many cancer patients rationalize that although they are physically changed, they possess unique, individual qualities; their courage, wit, intelligence, and warmth are still there, and they are still lovable and attractive. But words and self-encouragement don't seem to do the trick. What does work, according to cancer patients, is having your partner treat you like a whole and attractive person. Then you know everything will be OK. However, you have to give him or her a chance. You must be willing to expose yourself to the possibility that your partner actually will have the reaction you most fear.

If your partner has taken the lead and reestablished the sexual relationship, you don't have a problem. But if not, although it may frighten you silly, you can give the signal that you are interested in the same intimacy as before the illness—even come right out and ask for it.

With the right response, your sexual life together can return to where it was before, or close to it. But if you don't take the initiative, your partner may remain too worried to ask you, and intimacy might be indefinitely delayed or forgotten.

Suppose, however, that your "significant other" *is* actually put off by the change in your body. You should know this, too, and you should realize that this could change with the passage of time. There is no alternative but to be patient for a reasonable period.

If your partner's feelings don't change, what then? The answer, I'm afraid, is that I don't know. At The Wellness Community, results have varied from divorce or separation to acceptance of the changed relationship. That's just the way it is.

At this point, it's appropriate to mention that some sexual problems brought about by cancer are so complex as to require the help of a trained therapist, such as a psychiatrist, psychologist, clinical social worker, or marriage and family therapist. Sometimes your physician can help. As *Sexual Side Effects of Cancer* advises, "It's reasonable to say to your doctor: 'I have concerns about sex. Is this a problem you can help me with or can you send me to someone else?'"

PHYSICAL INABILITY

When temporary or permanent bodily changes make it difficult or impossible to receive or give pleasure as you did before, other methods must be found. Some solutions are described in *Sexual Side Effects of Cancer*:

> Genital intercourse is only one way of expressing physical love. People find that using hands, thumbs, fingers, tongues, lips, mouth, and anal areas may provide exciting and pleasurable alternatives to penile-vaginal intercourse. Intra-thigh and intra-mammary (placing the penis between the thighs or between the breasts) may also be an option. All these options are "normal sex."... Masturbation is a form of sexual activity that can be a satisfactory alternative form of gratification when sexual inter-

course is not possible or not desired.... Some women have found that mechanical vibrators can be
used, either by themselves or along with other sexual activities with their partners.

But nothing can take place without communication.
Everything changes when partners tell each other what
gives them the most pleasure. And partners can guide each
other's hands to the areas of pleasure and indicate how hard
or soft they want the pressure there to be. That's communication, too.

FEAR OF "CATCHING" CANCER

The final observation relates to the fear of "catching" cancer
through sexual contact. It may be expressed in thoughts like,
"I know this is irrational, but way down deep, I wonder if I
can catch cancer from my partner—maybe from his sperm, or
from saliva," or "from her secretions."

This gut feeling can severely inhibit sexual contact. Unless you overcome these fears through the knowledge that
there is no evidence that cancer is contagious or transmit-
table by sexual activity, your sex life will come to a total
halt— and for a meaningless reason.

---

45. Your partner's need for intimacy

❧

Recently, I asked the partners of cancer patients what emotions they were experiencing related to sex. The emotion that
surfaced most often was guilt over their need for sex while
their partner was so ill.

But just as it's true that life for the cancer patient does not end with the diagnosis, life for his or her partner also continues. The hormones that were bubbling before are still active. The desires may go into hiding for a while, but they soon emerge as strong as ever. The desire for affection and intimacy, even after a partner develops cancer, is nothing to feel guilty about.

The partners also confessed to guilt after having intercourse, convinced that their partner did it just to oblige them. After discussion, however, the group agreed upon a number of conclusions, including:

- Guilt related to one's sexual needs after one's partner is diagnosed with cancer is unrealistic and unnecessary.

- Most partners of cancer patients believe that the cancer patient should make a reasonable effort to meet his or her partner's sexual needs.

- In many instances, the sexual needs of both parties are unknown because both parties fail to discuss the problem and are left guessing how the other feels.

- With tenderness and concern, the needs of both parties can be met.

- Communication will clarify, if not solve, most of these problems.

46. Special sexual and intimacy problems confronting singles

❧

Being single and without a committed sexual partner creates additional concerns for a person who has cancer.

- How do you tell a potential sexual partner that you have cancer?
- How do you tell a potential partner that the disease or its treatment has left you with only one breast, with an ostomy bag, or unable to have an erection?
- When do you make these facts known?

The mere fact that you have cancer will be enough to make it impossible for some people to have a long-term relationship with you. They just aren't going to let themselves fall in love with someone who is facing cancer-related problems, and both of you should know that as soon as possible. While you should probably not open a conversation by saying, "Hello, my name is John (or Jane) Smith and I have cancer," you should make the fact known as soon as you see the relationship starting to move in the direction of permanency, because sooner or later, the information is going to come out.

This early communication is only fair to the other party, and it will also protect you from being hurt more deeply than need be. If the other person is going to move away, let it be before you become more involved. All kinds of rationalizations can be made for withholding the information, but the consensus is "the earlier, the better."

The question of how you convey the information has only one answer: Say it straight out. For instance, "John (Jane), I find that I'm looking forward to seeing you more and

more, and it seems to me that you are becoming more interested in me. Because of that, I want you to know that I have
(or have had) cancer." The conversation will go on from
there.

As far as bodily changes are concerned, your potential
partner is going to find out about them as soon as intimacy
begins. *Don't let the discovery of this bodily change come as
a shock at a time of arousal.* If he is reaching for a breast
that isn't there, or she suddenly realizes you are wearing
some type of ostomy bag, your partner may say or exclaim
something for which you both will be sorry. Tell your partner
about the bodily change under neutral, non-aroused circumstances so that he or she will have time to ask questions and
accept the information. If that information makes the relationship impossible, you'd better find out—and the sooner, the
better.

V

CONFRONTING CONFUSING ISSUES

47. Whom should I tell that I have cancer?

❧

Tell everyone you want to know, and don't tell anyone you don't want to know. However, remember that keeping cancer secret is difficult, particularly if your appearance changes.

A more pertinent question is, Why don't you want some people to know? If they knew, would you lose your job or some other benefit? If that's the case, the secret is well kept.

You might want to refer back to the discussion in chapter 40 about keeping secrets in groups. The basic suggestion is the same: Don't use up more energy keeping secrets than you have to.

48. How should I relate to my doctor?

❧

This relationship is of exquisite importance to the patient. A good relationship enhances the quality of life and the possibility of recovery, while a bad one impedes it and makes life more difficult for everyone. In this chapter, we'll consider the issue of the patient-physician relationship from the patient's point of view.

Herbert Benson, M.D., underscored the importance of the patient-physician relationship when he wrote that the placebo effect (the body's ability to heal itself) works when three elements are present: "One, the belief and expectation of the patient; two, the belief and expectation of the physician; and three, *the interaction between the patient and the physician.*"

Thus, the quality of the interaction between the patient and the physician is not a matter to be left to chance. But a rocky beginning for this relationship is not uncommon, because the cancer patient's first reaction after diagnosis is typically shock and disbelief, followed by the "why me" syndrome, and then unreasoning anger. At that time, what the patient wants to hear more than anything else is that the diagnosis is a mistake, or at least that the illness will be of brief duration and leave no lasting effects. And who but the physician is the one who must disappoint the patient in this regard, while prescribing medications, procedures, and tests that can have unpleasant side effects. As a result, it's not unusual for the patient's anger to land on the physician, setting up a delicate and sometimes uncomfortable situation.

Although a great majority of physicians respond as caring fellow human beings, there are a few who do eliminate all hope, who are distant, who won't answer questions, and who treat the patient like a not-too-bright employee. Even when the physician is sensitive and caring, a doctor-patient dance always ensues, with the physician doing the leading. If the physician can direct the patient's anger at the real enemy— the disease—the doctor and patient can fight that enemy as a team. If, on the other hand, the doctor is less than adroit at the psychological task of helping the patient, the relationship can be forever marred, much to the patient's detriment.

In the early stages of the illness, all of the responsibility falls upon the physician, who is at no risk, is the professional, and has been in similar circumstances many times before. The doctor should be prepared for the reactions of the patient, and should have developed some way to transmit information to a frightened, bewildered person in a manner that is supportive, hopeful, positive, yet accurate. Any physician who acts and speaks in an uncaring or insensitive way that strips the patient of all hope is either not aware of the crucial importance of the patient-physician relationship or just doesn't care. Fortunately, such behavior is by far the exception.

Of course, a medical degree does not bestow sainthood or unlimited patience, and a physician cannot be expected to act forever as a caring friend and confidant to an overly demanding, hostile, and angry patient. As in every interaction, the patient-physician connection must be a two-way street.

In many respects, the patient-physician relationship is the same as a business relationship with any independent contractor, such as a lawyer, accountant, plumber, or mechanic; each is paid for doing the best he or she can to accomplish the desired results. But physicians are special in several ways. They help us maintain or regain our most precious possession, our health. In no other situation does the independent contractor have so much responsibility. In no other situation is it quite so important that his or her advice and ministrations be correct, and that errors of both judgment and performance be avoided. In few other situations is so much training required and so many obligations placed on the independent contractor.

One of those obligations is to instill confidence and a feeling of security in the patient, while not appearing too authoritarian or remote. This is a very difficult role to play, and woe to the physician who fails us in any way or does not perform as expected.

CHOOSING AND USING YOUR DOCTOR

Because a good relationship with the right physician is of overriding importance to the cancer patient, the Patient Active commits as much time and energy as is necessary—and sometimes it takes quite a bit—to attain such a relationship. Choosing a medically competent physician is the first step. In most cases, this is done primarily by recommendation and reputation.

The next step is ensuring that the relationship is, at the very least, cordial. The variations of the patient-physician relationship are as numerous and as varied as there are patients and doctors. Some patients want every bit of information they can get. Others want to hear nothing but instructions. Some want to know what the alternatives are and want to make the final decisions themselves. Some want the doctor to decide what's best. Some consider waiting in a waiting room an acceptable inconvenience, while others find it intolerable. Some want to ask questions, write down answers, and have other people in the examining room. Others don't.

Physicians are also different. Most look forward to having the patient act as a partner. Others, because of temperament or training, can only interact with patients as a parental figure.

In a paper discussing the importance of a good patient-physician relationship, Howard Leventhal, Ph.D., and his colleagues at the University of Wisconsin discussed the necessity that each clearly understand the expectations of the other:

> Both patient and physician have specific expectations of and preferences for the type of relationship they will enjoy and the outcome they expect from their interaction. The expectations held by each party may differ considerably, and these differences may go unrecognized. Since the relationship places the physician in general control of the interaction, the substance of the relationship is likely to conform more closely to his or her expectations. Thus, to the extent that the patient's and physician's expectations differ, the patient may ultimately be unhappy with the care and may be less likely to remain in and comply with the treatment.

A frank discussion is therefore indicated, preferably after a reasonable breaking-in period during which you have become aware of what your needs are and how your doctor is responding to them. But don't put off the discussion too long;

you don't want too much time to pass while the problems of cancer are exacerbated by petty annoyances.

Very often, it is difficult for the patient to start the conversation with the doctor. After all, physicians have always been authority figures. But start it anyway. With very few exceptions, your physician is as anxious to have the conversation as you are. The dialogue should continue as long as necessary and recur when any part of the relationship appears unsatisfactory.

The discussion can range from how decisions regarding treatment will be made to questions as mundane as whether you and the physician will be on a first-name basis. If he calls you John, you call him Frank; it has become unthinkable for the 42-year-old physician to call his 65-year-old patient by her first name and expect her to call him "doctor."

When you understand the expectations of your physician, you can determine what accommodations you should make if those expectations do not coincide with yours. If your needs as a patient conflict seriously with the doctor's style, consider whether it's in your best interest to find another physician. Most people find it difficult and sometimes embarrassing to leave a physician. Although this rather drastic step should be taken only after serious consideration, it's not impossible or unthinkable. If the situation is irreparable, it's appropriate.

Often cancer patients are treated by a group of physicians that may include an oncologist, radiologist, surgeon, and/or some other specialist, along with the family doctor. One of the patient's most frequent complaints is that no one is in charge—each physician acts almost independently—and there is no one to whom the patient can talk to get *all* the information needed to make a decision. Therefore, it's important that you try to get one of the doctors to be the coordinator of the team and the repository of all information.

When you are satisfied that you have found the right physician(s), the next step is nurturing the relationship. It does not have to blossom into a full-blown friendship for it to be effective and efficient. It is only necessary that it be agreeable.

One of our participants summed up his perception of his role in this relationship as follows:

> As a cancer patient, I cannot think of anyone whose approval I am more interested in than my oncologist's. I want him to think of me as a decent, reasonable man who wants to recover more than anything else in the world. While he may not look forward to the day he is scheduled to see me, I wouldn't want him to dread it.
>
> In order to be worthy of my doctor's respect, I am, within my own capabilities, courteous, friendly, and considerate of his time. I am careful that my demands on him are reasonable. I try to be constantly aware that he is not a God who can cure me with a wave of his hand, that he has other patients, and that his entire life does not revolve around me alone.

One admonition: don't ask for a prognosis or inquire about longevity statistics unless you are actually ready to hear the answer. Most physicians refuse to make any prediction about longevity because they just don't know what an individual's life expectancy will be. If hard-pressed, they will discuss the statistics but will also describe patients who substantially outlived the statistics or who recovered completely.

Also, decide with your doctor how much you want to know and what part you want to play in the decision-making process. Make sure that those issues are clear between you and that you both agree.

Not long ago I had a discussion with about twenty participants. From that dialogue, it became apparent that most of them had complete confidence in their physicians and were generally happy with their relationship. But there were also some horror stories, particularly about physicians stripping the patient of hope.

This interchange raised the question of what a cancer patient could reasonably expect from a physician. I decided to meet with and ask the experts, the oncologists on The Wellness Community's Professional Advisory Board: Laurence Heifetz, then co-director of the Department of Oncology at Cedars-Sinai Medical Center; Daniel Lieber, then director of the Oncology Unit at Santa Monica Hospital and Research Institute; Frank Rosenfelt, an oncologist in private practice in Los Angeles; Richard Steckel, director of the Jonsson Comprehensive Cancer Center at UCLA; and Michael B. Van Scoy-Mosher, an oncologist in private practice in West Los Angeles.

At that meeting, the oncologists concurred that some patients, while receiving proper medical care, had relationships with their physicians that were not the most conducive to recovery, and that many patients believed that insensitive treatment by their doctors was normal. Eventually, we prepared a statement and tested it by distribution to 300 cancer patients. It is designed to help you judge whether your relationship with your own oncologist is all it should be. You might show it to your physician and discuss it with him or her.

THE WELLNESS COMMUNITY PATIENT/ONCOLOGIST STATEMENT

The effective treatment of serious illness requires a considerable effort by both the patient and the physician. A clear understanding by both of us as to what each of us can realistically and reasonably expect of the other will do much to enhance the outlook. I am giving this "statement" to you as one step in making our relationship as effective and productive as possible. It might be helpful if you would read this statement and, if you think it appropriate, discuss it with me.

As your physician, I will make every effort to:

1. Provide you with the care most likely to be beneficial to you.

2. Inform and educate you about your situation and the various treatment alternatives. How detailed an explanation is given will be dependent upon your specific desires.

3. Encourage you to ask questions about your illness and its treatment. I will answer your questions as clearly as possible. I will also attempt to answer the questions asked by your family; however, my primary responsibility is to you, and I will discuss your medical situation only with those people authorized by you.

4. Remain aware that all major decisions about the course of your care shall be made by you. However, I will accept the responsibility for making certain decisions if you want me to.

5. Assist you to obtain other professional opinions if you desire, or if I believe it to be in your best interests.

6. Relate to you as one competent adult to another, always attempting to consider your emotional, social, and psychological needs as well as your physical needs.

7. Spend a reasonable amount of time with you on each visit unless required by something urgent to do otherwise, and give you my undivided attention during that time.

8. Honor all appointments unless required by something urgent to do otherwise.

9. Return phone calls as promptly as possible, especially those you indicate are urgent.

10. Make test results available promptly if you desire such reports.

11. Provide you with any information you request

concerning my professional training, experience, philosophy, and fees.

12. Respect your desire to try treatments that might not be conventionally accepted. However, I will give you my honest opinion about such unconventional treatments.

13. Maintain my active support and attention throughout the course of the illness.

I hope that you as the patient will make every effort to:

1. Comply with our agreed-upon treatment plan.

2. Be as candid as possible with me about what you need and expect from me.

3. Inform me if you desire another professional opinion.

4. Inform me of all forms of therapy you are involved with.

5. Honor all appointment times unless required by something urgent to do otherwise.

6. Be as considerate as possible of my need to adhere to a schedule to see other patients.

7. Attempt to make all phone calls to me during regular working hours. Call on nights and weekends only when absolutely necessary.

8. Attempt to coordinate the requests of your family and confidants, so that I do not have to answer the same questions about you to several different persons.

GUIDELINES FOR VISITS WITH PHYSICIANS

Now that you know what five prominent oncologists believe you can expect, the following quidelines may be useful in your relationship with and visits to your doctor, helping you:

- Understand the instructions given to you more thoroughly and comply with them more precisely.

• Get the information you need quickly.

• Have greater peace of mind because you will be aware of the procedures being used and the hoped-for results.

• Have more confidence in your physician because of his or her ability and willingness to explain the plan of treatment in language understandable to you.

The recommendations are as follows:

• Before the visit, prepare a written list of the questions you want to ask your doctor. This will save office time and assure that all your questions are asked.

• For the same reasons, before the visit, prepare a written list of the information you want the doctor to know.

• If you don't understand something your doctor says, say so. If you don't speak up, you may follow the wrong advice or take an improper amount of medication.

• Take someone with you when you visit your doctor. Your friend will not be as stressed as you and will be able to listen to and understand the doctor with greater objectivity.

• Get a second opinion when a major course of action is contemplated.

• If you want to, decide with your physician between the various alternatives presented. Such a protocol is becoming the norm, according to Irving L. Janis, Ph.D., of Yale University:

During recent decades, there has been a marked change in the way people in our society, including health experts, view the role of the patient. No

longer are patients seen as passive recipients of
health care who are expected to do willingly whatever the doctor says. Rather, they are increasingly
regarded as active decision-makers, making a series
of crucial choices that can markedly affect the kind
of treatments they receive and the outcome.

You should do everything in your power to ensure that
your relationship with your physician is as trouble-free as
possible. Make certain that any problems between you and
your doctor are not your fault, and then discuss any problem
areas with him. If that doesn't work, find a new physician.

---

49. I want things to return to exactly the way they were before the diagnosis. Is that possible?

❧

No person can come through an experience as traumatic as
cancer without changing. Furthermore, I'm not sure you'll
want to when you think about it. When I hear cancer patients
say that's what they want, my first reaction is to visualize the
many people I know to whom cancer is a memory and who
have no doubt that their lives are more fulfilling because of
their experience with cancer.

Many learned to love in a different and better way, learned
what is important in life, learned that success comes in many
different forms, not just money and power. They learned how
powerful they really are ("If I can come through cancer, I
can fight back from anything"). They learned that they get
most pleasure out of helping others. Of course, many of them

have physical reminders of the illness that they would be happy to do without. But such change is a fact of life with which they live.

I watched many cancer patients change careers, reconcile with parents and children, divorce spouses, go back to school, take up art, give up art, become more assertive, become less aggressive. Sometimes the changes don't last and they revert to their old ways. They become the same workaholics they were before, or they once again become the compliant, submissive, "too good to be true" person everyone loves. Some forget the lessons they learned unless some physical symptom raises the specter of the illness's return, or something else reminds them of their bout with cancer.

Sometimes they even resume smoking, or drinking more than is good for them. Raymond, for example, was told by his physician at the time of the diagnosis of Type B lymphoma that his drinking might have had something to do with the onset of the illness, and that it certainly wasn't doing him any good. He immediately gave up alcohol and began to work diligently as a Patient Active. Within a relatively short time, during which he became completely bald from chemotherapy, his physician told him that he was fully recovered. The chemo stopped and his hair grew back.

Six months later, Raymond was back, once again bald. With the regrowth of his hair, he had forgotten all the lessons he had learned from cancer and started to drink heavily again. The symptoms reappeared, and he is fighting to recover once more, off the stuff now—hopefully forever.

While some ex-cancer patients forget the lessons that cancer taught them, those who spend their time helping other patients remember the lessons very well. They relearn them every time they tell their stories to newcomers and watch them learn the same lessons. They don't fool themselves into believing that cancer never happened.

Finally, one problem faced by every person I have ever met who has had cancer is the fear of recurrence. While cancer patients are going through the process of fighting for recovery, and even after they have been without symptoms for many years, every headache that would have been ignored prior to the diagnosis becomes worrisome as a possible new site of cancer. Every backache formerly accepted as a chronic condition now becomes a harbinger of the spread or return of the illness. But when it is discovered that these fears and apprehensions are shared by all cancer patients, the fear abates. It never seems to disappear, but it abates.

So the questions become: Do you *really* want to return to exactly the way you were before the diagnosis? Do you *really* want to forget that you ever had cancer? I'm not sure you do.

---

50. Are there actually benefits to having cancer?

Cancer is a difficult way to gain anything, and if given the choice, I'm sure you'd select other ways to reap such benefits. But they exist nonetheless.

One benefit of having cancer is that it may teach you how to enjoy one day at a time. One woman described the lesson she learned this way:

> I myself find it hard to believe what I am going to say, but there are some ways in which I'm glad I have cancer. I spent all of my life being a legal librarian, and that's all I ever was. Although I have a husband and children, now grown, I wasn't a mother and a wife, I was a legal librarian.
>
> When cancer came along, I started to look at my children and husband as precious. Now when

we're together, I know I love them and they fill me with joy. In a strange way, their concern about my well-being also makes me very happy. I'm not sure I would ever have learned to love in any other way.

One woman with colon cancer participated in Wellness Community groups for more than three years, fighting cancer all the way. She has been in complete remission for a year, and about six months ago she moved to the East. After describing how well she felt, she wrote:

> For about three weeks after the diagnosis, although I was still feeling pretty good, I was in a complete funk. All I could think about was all the people and things I was going to miss when I died. I couldn't talk to anyone without crying. Then one day, while looking at but not seeing a television program, it came to me in a flash that I was already missing all of the good things in life. And I realized that everything in life was good, and that it was all passing me by without my even seeing it.
>
> I went into the room where my mother and father were sitting, and we all went out for sodas. From that minute on, I kept looking around and seeing all of the "good" things in life. Even when I was feeling sick from treatment, and believed I was going to die from cancer, I still realized that life was filled with things to do, places to go, and people to love.
>
> About two weeks ago, my new doctor told me that the cancer is all behind me. And now I'm even more thrilled with what I see, hear, and feel. I hope I never lose it. If I do, I want all of you to kick me you-know-where.

Another benefit of cancer is that it can free you to choose the options in life that lead to your being as happy as possible *now*. One of our participants, Edward, realized that:

Before the diagnosis, I was working ten to twelve hours a day with a coat and tie, under extreme pressure to try to do the job better than I did it the day before, and not liking it very much. Then all of a sudden I had cancer. Within days after the diagnosis, I said to myself, "Holy smoke! I don't have to do all of that anymore—I have cancer! I really should concentrate on getting better and enjoying life as it is." And I started to do just that.

Although I had to earn a living before I had cancer, I didn't have to relinquish all present joy. But I did. Before the diagnosis, I was forgoing present happiness for future happiness. Then cancer made me realize that the future might never come. Now, even though I've been symptom-free for quite a while, I still operate on the principle that the future may never come. Although I can't ignore it entirely, I can do everything possible to make the present happy, too.

Further insight into this subject comes from John, another Wellness Community participant. Three days before we spoke, John had received the news that his tumor, which had been doubling in size every two months for some time, showed signs of regressing. He said:

Now that it looks like I have a chance for recovery, I realize what freedom cancer brings. When you believe there's no chance of recovery, you are like a nine- or ten-year-old. As far as the future is concerned, there is none, and therefore you don't have to worry. All you have to concern yourself with is the present.

With the good news I just received, I feel my concern for the future sneaking back in. I can't continue to ignore it. Every action I now take must be weighed in terms of the effect it will have on my life somewhere down the road. There's a part of me that's ecstatic about the good news. But there's another part of me that hates to give up the freedom of living only in the present. However, I'll never forget the lesson I've learned. I'll never again let concern for the future make the present unpleasant.

I have also met many cancer patients who, with the onset of the illness, have felt compelled to renew and reestablish old, sometimes severed, relationships. Charlie, a 55-year-old widower with lung cancer, had not spoken to any of his four siblings for over thirty years. But almost immediately after the diagnosis, facing up to the fact that life does not go on forever, Charlie traveled to the East Coast and visited with his three brothers and sister for six weeks. He recalled:

> The reunion was the most emotional time of my life. We laughed, cried, hugged, and kissed, but what we did most in the beginning was just look at one another. For the first time in many years, I realized how much I love those people. And we could hardly remember what happened so many years ago that got in the way of that love.

Some three years later, Charlie's house is now hardly ever without a brother, a sister, a niece, or a nephew in it. "I've never been happier," said Charlie, "and if cancer hadn't come along and scared me out of my wits, I would have missed all this."

In such cases, of course, the family reaps the "benefits" of the disease as well. Consider Marci, whose father became ill with cancer. With some surprise in her voice, she recently recalled that one of her early impulses, after the shock and sorrow had worn off a little, was to call Carla, who had been her best friend in high school. The women had had a falling-out in college and hadn't talked to each other since, but, Marci explained, "knowing that I was soon to lose one important person in my life, I recognized how silly it was to permit pettiness or pride to deprive me of another important relationship before it came to its natural conclusion."

When Marci called Carla, who lived in another city, something they had both missed and longed for was rekindled. Their warmth and love for one another were reestablished.

Cancer, like other illnesses, can also bring what psychologists term secondary gains. This delicate issue can best be defined by the following question: Are there any benefits you are receiving from the illness that are, on an unconscious level, interfering with your desire to recover? The answer to that question is seldom an unequivocal "yes," but it can be a "maybe," and that "maybe" can be interfering with both your conscious and unconscious efforts to recover.

One of the more striking examples was Elaine, who had been married for four years. For some reason, the very thought of sleeping with her husband had become extremely unpleasant to her. She found that with the onset of breast cancer, she was relieved of that unwelcome "obligation." In her group, she discovered just how relieved she was at not having to perform or make lame excuses.

On an unconscious level, Elaine and many patients like her often realize that if and when they recover, they will have to give up their secondary gain. *On the unconscious level, they decide they would rather have cancer than forgo this "benefit."*

It is impossible to know whether the set of facts in Elaine's life played any part in the onset of her illness. But cancer did teach her that there are many other ways of handling an unpleasant situation—such as, in this case, candor, psychotherapeutic help, or divorce. It's also quite possible that in bringing the realization of her relief from the subconscious to the conscious, Elaine gained considerable stress reduction.

Other common types of secondary gains can be quite subtle. For instance, a wife with cancer may no longer have to do the ironing, a chore she hates, although she is really well enough to do it. Or a husband may not have to attend social affairs he despises, even though he really could. Or an employee with cancer may be able to shift much of the burden of his job to fellow workers, although he is actually still capable of doing much of that work.

So the advice of this chapter is to make sure you take advantage of all the positive benefits that come with cancer and catalogue them either mentally or in writing, so that they will be forever part of the life experiences that guide you. Then ask yourself, your group, or your friends if you are enjoying a secondary gain that, on an unconscious level, may be more important to you than recovery. Additionally, you might explore whether you are using the illness to get away with anything or to get out of doing something you're healthy enough to do. But be careful. Don't push yourself too hard. Your primary job is to get physically well, not to improve your psychological condition or win a popularity contest.

---

51. Is it best for me to be brave and cheerful always?

❧

A woman named Marie recently described our first meeting to a large group we were both addressing as follows: I had been fighting cancer alone for more than two years, and I was becoming very tired. My doctor, aware of how draining the illness and the treatments were on me both mentally and physically, advised me to investigate The Wellness Community. But a year before I had joined a group of cancer patients and the incessant complaining had been so depressing that I dropped out after two meetings.

However, one Sunday morning, when things weren't going well, I went to The Wellness Community and talked to Harold Benjamin about the Patient Active concept and decided to come to a Sharing Group and soon became an active participant in every part of the program.

To make clear the point of this anecdote, let me describe our meeting from *my* point of view. My first impression of Marie was of a very attractive woman walking unsteadily with a cane, but whose unsure gait was overshadowed by her spirit. This spirit seemed to give a rosy glow to everything around her. Although she tells me now she was depressed, I never knew it.

Later, whenever Marie was in the facility, I always looked forward to her visits. But as time passed, I saw her less and less frequently, although she was still coming to the Community as often as before. Wondering why, I asked the facilitator of Marie's group to ask Marie about it. Her explanation:

> Being with Harold became just too hard. He always expected me to be cheerful and energetic, when sometimes I just wanted to be tired old me. But I knew he wouldn't like me that way, so I just stayed away.

I learned from that experience that many cancer patients, believing that their friends can't face knowing just how frightened, tired, or ill they really feel, determine to act brave and cheerful all of the time. Their friends, in turn, believe that the only "right" way to act with a cancer patient is to always be brave and cheerful themselves. And it doesn't work.

There are very few relationships that can survive the always-brave-and-cheerful syndrome, and such forced gaiety must place a tremendous strain on the immune system.

In looking back at my friendship with Marie, I can see how I contributed to her strain. Whenever I talked about Marie, I used her as an example. I never failed to mention how her cheerfulness brightened my day. So don't do it. Act brave and cheerful when you feel brave and cheerful *or* when you think that acting brave and cheerful is in your best interests. And when you don't—don't.

At this point, as you try to decide how best to participate in your fight for recovery, you may notice what appears to be a contradiction. In chapter 31, I advised you to "act as if" you are always cheerful, while here, I tell you to act as you feel. Both suggestions are merely choices you can make to fit your particular situation—not instructions.

So think about your reactions, and don't react in a particular way just because you think that's what others expect of you. Do what you think is best for you. And know that you have a choice.

And the same advice goes for friends and relatives, too. You don't have to be brave and cheerful all the time, either, and don't let the cancer patient think you expect this from him or her all the time. Once you stop expecting, you can start relating.

VI
FAMILY AND FRIENDS ASK

❧

52. What do I say to a cancer patient?

೮

This question is asked over and over by almost everyone who discovers that a friend or relative has cancer. We aren't usually frightened or intimidated by a friend who is recovering from heart bypass surgery or fighting off the effects of another disease. It takes very little psychological effort to visit him, and we know exactly how to act and precisely what to say.

But when the illness is cancer, most of us have to fight against all our impulses and force ourselves to visit the patient. Somehow, we don't know how to act or what to say, and we know that any conversation will be strained and difficult. So we stay away, and the cancer patient feels abandoned. Even when we are with the patient, we are so concerned about saying the "wrong" thing that the conversation is limited to the most innocuous types of interchange, and again the patient feels abandoned. Aware of how uncomfortable friends are in her presence, she too avoids such meetings. That's called reclusiveness.

In preparing this chapter, I called together twenty-five participants of The Wellness Community and posed the following questions: "As a cancer patient, how do you want your friends and relatives to talk to you? What do you want them to say?"

Their advice can be summed up the following guidelines.

1. Be natural. Treat the cancer patient as much as possible as you did before the diagnosis. (This one suggestion really says it all. What follows is amplification and explanation.)

2. Don't be afraid to talk directly with the patient about cancer and how it is affecting him. If he doesn't feel like talking about it, he'll tell you; asking about it lets him know you're not too frightened to hear his feelings.

3. Maintain regular contact with the patient and include her in conversations about what's going on in your life, as well as in hers. She wants to feel connected with the well world, and she depends on you for that.

4. Don't be afraid to touch and hug the patient. He feels especially vulnerable about this, because he feels unlovable a lot of the time.

5. Don't pity the patient! That is the most awful feeling of all, and it doesn't help.

6. Don't tell her horror stories about cancer or any other disease.

7. Do tell him about any success stories you hear. They fuel his hope and belief in the possibility of his own recovery.

8. Be of as much practical help as you can to make the patient's life easier. Just as important, it lets her know that you care about her.

9. Refrain from well-intentioned advice, unless asked for it. The patient's health-care team guides him, and your suggestions only confuse and irritate him. On the other hand, he welcomes articles and books that he can look at on his own and form his own opinions about.

10. Celebrate any and all milestones along the way with the patient. Holidays and completions of treatment mean a lot to her and are more meaningful when shared with those she loves and cherishes most.

11. Don't forget that he wants to be part of your life and that he wants to laugh with you, just as before he became ill.

12. Don't set up a we/they situation. The patient is

still your friend or relative; the diagnosis didn't change this.

13. Don't be so sure that the patient is doomed. There are millions of *ex*-cancer patients.

Some cancer patients said they really don't want their family or friends to talk about the disease—they feel more "normal" if they are not reminded of it. But I believe these patients are in the minority. Most say they do want people to talk about it with them. Cancer is frightening enough, but when the subject is avoided, it becomes ominous. Having others indicate that they are willing to talk at any time about any aspect of the experience diminishes the cancer patient's fear, because it indicates that the illness is not so frightening as to be unmentionable.

One woman told about a childhood friend who didn't come to see her after learning she had cancer:

> She was afraid she'd cry when we got together. But we could have cried together. I would have understood and wanted that to happen. Her staying away hurt, and added to my feeling unlovable and untouchable.

Cancer patients want you to be direct so that they know what you are willing to talk about. A vague question like "How do you feel?" leaves them wondering whether it is merely a normal salutation or whether the friend actually wants to open a conversation about the illness. They prefer a more specific question; for example, "How is your treatment going?" If the cancer patient doesn't want to talk about the illness, he or she will let you know.

Some patients want to be asked questions about how cancer has changed their lives and values, but only after the treatment has progressed and their conditions have stabilized. Such questions give them a chance to express how their experience has helped them appreciate what is really important in life. Others don't want to talk about psychological matters to friends. They only want to talk about recovering and making plans for the future.

There is one topic cancer patients never tire of hearing about, and that is *ex*-cancer patients. And the more, the merrier. "What I want most to hear about are people for whom cancer is a memory," said one participant. "When I hear about cancer patients who have recovered, it gives me hope that I can get better, too."

"If you have had cancer and have recovered—tell me," said another participant. "If you haven't had cancer but know someone who has and has recovered, tell me about him."

Several of the cancer patients complained that friends sometimes say things like, "Don't worry, you'll have the surgery, radiation, and chemotherapy, and you'll be OK," as if the illness were a bad cold or an inflamed appendix. "This type of statement makes me feel like a child patted on the head," said one participant. "It doesn't reflect how fearsome this whole experience is and how uncertain the outcome of treatment really is."

She added that she wanted her friends and relatives to acknowledge the seriousness of her situation and to be with her to deal with the crisis together. "What I found most comforting was when I heard my husband and adult kids tell me that we would work together to find our way through this challenge. The worst moments were when I felt alone with the burden of what to do with my overwhelming feelings of insecurity, terror, and despair."

Another participant said, "All of us want to be loved and needed, but when you have cancer, you are exceptionally needy. You need people to show that they like, value, and care about you. Friends and family can do that by taking you out to lunch, driving you to appointments, or bringing dinner in from time to time."

Hearing about your life is important, too. Cancer patients want to share feelings in a balanced way, so that they don't always feel that they're the patient and you're the well person. Keeping conversations light at times and talking about things other than cancer help the patient feel part of the world of the living, rather than "just one big cancer symptom," as one participant put it.

One type of communication that everyone considers rude, overbearing, and depressing is the "helpful" suggestion. One participant said, "Don't tell me what I should or shouldn't do. These well-intentioned remarks—like 'You shouldn't focus on your cancer so much,' 'You shouldn't eat such and such,' 'You should push yourself more'—which are often contradictory since they come from different sources—are irritating, even though the motivation behind them is supportive."

Whatever the content and whatever the motivation, any message that starts with a "should" from anyone but a physician seems like another effort to deprive the patient of one more area of control. If the cancer patient asks your advice and you think you may have an answer, offer it. But otherwise, hold back. Cancer patients are already getting about as much advice as they can handle.

Having friends and relatives recognize the achievement of goals adds a positive aspect to the lives of cancer patients. Celebrations after chemo treatments and for birthdays are especially important, since the thought often crosses the patient's mind that she may not reach the next birthday. Making an occasion out of these events gives everyone joy and a window into the future. As one woman put it:

> I had my fiftieth birthday in the middle of my chemotherapy, and my friends gave me a big party. I loved it! I wasn't in very good shape, but I did as much as I could—and enjoyed it. I was so happy to see that they were all there, and to realize that I actually gotten to my fiftieth birthday.

Finally, I have learned over the years that there are occasions, most of which arise when the news about the illness has not been good or the symptoms are particularly ominous, where the only appropriate reaction is to just listen. Words of cheerful encouragement are sometimes out of place. Silent attentiveness indicates not only understanding, but also a willingness to be one with the speaker, to share her emotions and by sharing them reduce her burden to some small degree. The decision as to when silence is the best communication requires sensitivity and a careful reading of the desires and needs of the cancer patient. To attempt to persuade that all is, or soon will be, well, when that eventuality is unlikely, can introduce an unbridgeable gulf between those who are ill and those who are well.

---

53. I don't have cancer. Is there anything I can do to make the possibility of developing cancer more unlikely?

આ

The following suggestions are gleaned from conversations with many cancer patients in which they indicated what they would have done in an attempt to avoid cancer, if they had known before diagnosis what they know now. They did not consider issues such as smoking, nutrition, or exercise.

1. Learn as much as you can about what cancer is and how it is caused, so that you will be aware of those activities that may be dangerous and those that may be beneficial (see chapters 2 through 11).

2. Since you know now that stress can be physically harmful, you might want to consider how best to alter your behavior or your lifestyle so that you encounter as little stress as possible, and that you take such steps as are available to see to it that your reactions to stressors are as bland and/or as short a duration as possible (see chapters 31 and 32).

3. Many cancer patients who consider directed visualization (see chapter 32) an integral part of their fight for recovery express regret that they weren't aware of this technique before the diagnosis. It would have provided them another method of counteracting the harmful physical results of negative stress. You might consider using directed visualization in the hope that it may help your immune system remain as strong as possible.

4. Since forced aloneness is unhealthy (see chapter 25), be sure you have as many social contacts as you are comfortable with. And remember that laughter and joy may enhance your body's power to fight off illness.

VII

ABOUT THE
WELLNESS COMMUNITY

54. The evolution of The Wellness Community

In this book, you have learned how to benefit from the concepts developed at The Wellness Community. But unless you understand their genesis, the recommendations made here will be as mysterious as the procedures and medicines prescribed by physicians, and just as difficult to modify to fit individual requirements and lifestyles. This chapter will briefly describe the evolution of The Wellness Community program.

I came to the "science" of the psychological aspects of cancer therapy through a rather circuitous route. For thirty years (1950 – 1980) I practiced law in New York City and Beverly Hills, and for some of those years (1966 – 1975) I was involved in Synanon as a "square." ("Square" in this context is a nonderogatory word for someone who does not have a problem with drugs.)

Synanon was then a residential drug rehabilitation program founded in the early 1960s in Santa Monica, California, where drug abusers came to "kick the habit" and to recover from the psychological addiction to drugs. They lived, worked, and played together in the Synanon facility and were required to attend several therapeutic groups with other residents each week. My family and I were residents of Synanon for five years.*

Synanon participants became part of a therapeutic community, which is a program based on the premise that people fighting to recover from a malady can benefit greatly on a psychological level from long-term intimate contact with others facing the same or similar problems, and from continuous exposure to therapeutic groups.

---

*In late 1975, there was much adverse publicity about Synanon. By then, my wife and I had already left.

At Synanon, I became aware of the tremendous power for psychological good that can come from a therapeutic community. And when my wife had a mastectomy, I learned how healthy such a community can be for someone with a serious illness. Harriet didn't become a second-class citizen in Synanon because she had cancer. Her friends there didn't look upon her as "dying." To them, she was the same Harriet Benjamin she had been before the operation. She encountered none of the rejection so many cancer patients face daily. She had all of her friends beside her supporting her fight to regain her health.

As soon as she was able, Harriet went back to performing the executive functions for which she was responsible before the surgery. She received love, support, and encouragement but experienced no knee-jerk sympathy, no pity, no reluctance to be with her because of the illness.

There is no doubt in my mind that all of this support improved the quality of Harriet's life. I also can't help but believe that it had something to do with the fact that since her mastectomy, Harriet has been leading a very active, symptom-free life. This experience had a deep and lasting effect on me. On some subconscious level, I learned that camaraderie, togetherness, and support can help people with serious illness. And when I later became familiar with the problems of cancer patients, this knowledge surfaced and gave rise to The Wellness Community concept of the Patient Active.

From my experience in Synanon, I learned the benefits that a therapeutic community can produce:

- It promotes a sense of belonging and friendship, which dissipates loneliness, adds joy and contentment to life, and modifies or eliminates insecurity and doubt about one's lovableness.

- The more we reveal about ourselves, the less time and energy we expend hiding parts of our personality that we perceive as unattractive.

- Most of the components of our personalities that we consider unique and terrible, and therefore deserving of secrecy, are shared by most other people.

- By revealing habit patterns that make us unhappy, we can learn to modify them.

- Such interaction can release stress in our lives.

- The energy conserved by such revelations can be better directed toward actions that make us happier.

- All of the above are amplified when the people we are with share a common purpose and desire a common result.

Almost everything recommended in this book, then, is based, in one way or another, on peer support, interpersonal relations, and camaraderie.

In 1976, I became friends with Hal Stone, a clinical psychologist and founder of The Center for the Healing Arts in West Los Angeles, which was created to train psychologists to treat individuals with life-threatening illnesses. From 1976 until 1981, I spent all my free time at the Center, or reading or going to lectures about the psychosocial aspects of serious illness. Most important, I also worked, played, and studied with many of the Center's clients, most of whom had cancer.

It was there that I observed that cancer patients have a tremendous need for support, hope, encouragement, and involvement in the fight for recovery; that they have become the modern-day lepers; and that most cancer patients are, to one extent or another, abandoned both physically and emotionally by their family and friends, just when they need support the most. I learned that in addition to financial problems and fear of suffering and death, the three most debilitating psychosocial problems that accompany cancer are feelings of helplessness and hopelessness, unwanted aloneness, and loss of control.

But I also learned that life does not end with the diagnosis of cancer and that there is always room for hope, joy, and involvement. I also discovered a wealth of material published over the last twenty years indicating strongly that an individual's efforts in the fight for recovery may enhance the possibility of recovery. This knowledge filled me with joy and hope.

I further learned that negative emotions can have negative physical effects, that positive emotions may be physically beneficial, and that there is scientific evidence to prove what I had intuited: that togetherness is good for people and unwanted aloneness can be physically and psychologically harmful.

Soon, all this began to merge into one cohesive concept. By 1981, it had become clear to me that what was needed was a program where cancer patients could receive the type of group therapy, peer support, and camaraderie I had learned about at Synanon, and the knowledge of how to deal with cancer from this psychological perspective I had learned about at The Center for the Healing Arts. I knew that such a program just might enhance the possibility of their recovery, and would certainly improve the quality of their lives.

While programs for cancer patients were springing up throughout the United States, each of them addressed itself only to a specific aspect of the problem. And there were no programs that included community—a place where cancer patients could meet, socialize, and give and receive peer support on a continuous basis. I knew that one had to be started, and I knew that I was the one to do it.

On January 1, 1982, I retired from the practice of law to devote full time to The Wellness Community. In those early days, I was joined by Shannon Behrens, a licensed therapist and former cervical cancer patient I had met at The Center for the Healing Arts.

Getting The Wellness Community off the ground was not easy. We found a facility in Santa Monica, but on our first day we had no backers or physicians on our side. All we had was an idea and six cancer patients. We started the first Participant Group under Shannon's direction.

After about six months, with no blemishes on our record and about thirty participants, we were invited to speak before more than twenty-five physicians from the Santa Monica area. After some direct grilling by several of the physicians about our motives and methods, the response was enthusiastically affirmative. More and more oncologists sent their patients to us. As we were helpful to more people with cancer, they told others about the program, who in turn also came to us.

Several prominent oncologists and psychologists involved with cancer patient care became members of our professional advisory board, and Norman Cousins agreed to be the honorary chairman of the board of directors.

After three years of operation, it became apparent to me that people with cancer everywhere could benefit by understanding and applying our concepts and procedures, even without a Wellness Community in their area. Recognizing that a book was needed, I set up many conversations with cancer patients and physicians to gather material. *From Victim to Victor* is the result.

---

55. A final message

❧

The choice is yours...to be a Patient Active or a patient passive.

If you have decided to be a Patient Active, you have chosen to be a vital, active part of the fight. You know that there are always alternatives and that you always have some choice in how you feel, how you act, and how you react. You know that there are very few situations where communication doesn't help. You have also learned what the myths about cancer are, and to the best of your ability, you have discarded them.

As a Patient Active, you understand that the mind and the body are actually one functioning unit, with every action of one affecting the other. You know that life doesn't end with the diagnosis of cancer and that cancer is not necessarily a sentence to death. You also know that if you fight for your recovery rather than sitting around waiting for someone to do it for you, you will improve the quality of your life, and this in and of itself may enhance the possibility of your recovery.

You are also doing your best to comply with the instructions of your physician. You are seeing to it that you are not alone more than you want to be. You are maintaining your social contacts. You have not given up more control of your life than you have to, and you are retaking control of areas where you had already given up unnecessarily.

You are using directed visualization because you want your immune system to be as strong as possible. In addition, you try to avoid triggering the fight-or-flight response when possible. You are using a support group if you can find one. You also are changing stressful situations by the "act as if" method and other techniques. You are doing all this work because you believe or hope that such efforts are important steps along your road to recovery.

Even if you are doing only some of these activities, you know that whatever you are doing is *right and proper for you,* and that there is no way you can be wrong in deciding how you will fight for recovery. You also know that you are not to blame for the onset of the disease, but that this does not mean you are powerless to fight for your recovery. You know too the outcome is not completely in your control; if the illness does not progress as you want it to, it's not your fault.

You've also learned that even with cancer, there is still room in life for joy, involvement, and, except in the most drastic of situations, intimacy and sexuality; that there is always room too for hope, no matter what the odds; that there are many lessons to be learned from cancer, although there must be better ways to learn them; and that cancer is not a curse but is a disease like any other. You know that many, many people recover from cancer, and you have met some of them through this book.

You also know that you and your doctor are a team fighting for your recovery, and that the medication and treatment you receive are part of that team. Most of all, you know that you have a choice: *You can be a Patient Active or a patient passive. And whatever you decide to do, there are untold numbers of people rooting for you and hoping for the best for you.*

BIBLIOGRAPHY

American Cancer Society. *Cancer Facts & Figures 1984.* New York: American Cancer Society, 1983.

Angell, Marcia. "Disease as a Reflection of the Psyche." *New England Journal of Medicine,* 312 (June 13, 1985): 1570-1572.

Bahnson, C. B. "Psychosomatic Issues in Cancer," in *The Psychosomatic Approach to Illness,* R. L. Gallon (ed.). New York: Elsevier Biomedical, 1982.

Benson, Herbert. "The Placebo Effect." *Harvard Medical School Health Letter,* August 1980, pp. 3-4.

Benson, Herbert. *The Relaxation Response.* New York: William Morrow & Co., 1975.

Berkman, Lisa F. and Breslow, Lester. *Health and Ways of Living.* New York: Oxford University Press, 1983.

Borysenko, Joan. "Psychoneuroimmunology: Behavioral Factors and the Immune Response." *ReVision,* 7 (Spring 1984): 56-65.

Braun, Bennett G. "Psychophysiologic Phenomena in Multiple Personality and Hypnosis." *American Journal of Clinical Hypnosis,* 26 (October 1983): 124-137.

Brown, Barbara. *New Mind, New Body.* New York: Irvington Publishers, 1986.

Cassileth, Barrie R.; Lusk, Edward J.; Miller, David S. et al. "Psychosocial Correlates of Survival in Advanced Malignant Disease." *New England Journal of Medicine,* 312 (June 13, 1985): 1551-1555.

Cousins, Norman. *Anatomy of an Illness.* New York: W. W. Norton & Co., 1979

Critelli, J. and Neumann, K. "The Placebo: Conceptual Analysis of a Construct in Transition." *American Psychologist,* 39: 32-39, January 1984.

Curt, Gregory. "Chemotherapy Treatment of Cancer." *Los Angeles Times,* March 21, 1987, Sec. 2, p. 2.

Derogatis, L. R.; Abeloff, M.D.; and Melisaratos, N. "Psychological Coping Mechanisms and Survival Time in Metastic Breast Cancer." *JAMA,* 242: 1504-1508, October 5, 1979.

Fiore, Neil A. "Fighting Cancer—One Patient's Perspective." *The New England Journal of Medicine,* 300: 284-289, February 8, 1979.

Fox, B. H. "Premorbid Psychological Factors as Related to Cancer Incidence." *Behavioral Medicine,* 1: 45-133, March 1978.

Friends Can Be Good Medicine. Sacramento: California Department of Mental Health, 1981.

Goldberg, Jane (ed.). *Psychotherapeutic Treatment of Cancer Patients.* New York: The Free Press, 1981.

Green, Elmer and Green, Alyce. *Beyond Biofeedback.* New York: Delacorte, 1977.

Hall, Howard. "Hypnosis and the Immune System: A Review with Implications for Cancer and the Psychology of Healing." *American Journal of Clinical Hypnosis,* 25 (October 1982): 92-103.

Holland, Jimmie. *Understanding the Cancer Patient.* New York: American Cancer Society, 1980.

Janis, Irving L. "The Patient as Decision Maker," in *Handbook of Behavioral Medicine,* W. Doyle Gentry (ed.). New York: The Guilford Press, 1984.

Kubler-Ross, Elisabeth. *On Death and Dying.* New York: Macmillan, 1970.

LeShan, L. and Worthington, R. E. "Some Recurrent Life History Patterns Observed in Patients with Malignant Disease." *Journal of Nervous and Mental Diseases,* 124: 460-465, May 1954.

Leventhal, Howard; Zimmerman, Rick; and Gutmann, Mary. "Compliance: A Self-Regulation Perspective," in *Handbook of Behavioral Medicine,* W. Doyle Gentry (ed.). New York: The Guilford Press, 1985.

Locke, Steven E. "Stress, Adaptation and Immunity: Studies in Humans." *General Hospital Psychiatry,* 4: 49-58, April 1982.

Lynch, James J. *The Broken Heart.* New York: Basic Books, 1977.

Menninger, R. W. "Psychiatry 1976: Time for a Holistic Medicine." *Annals of Internal Medicine,* 84 (May 1976): 5.

Merton, Robert K. "The Self-Fulfilling Prophecy." *Antioch Review,* 8: 193-210, June 1948.

Morra, Marion E. *Sexual Side Effects of Cancer.* Bethesda: National Cancer Institute, 1986.

O'Regan, Brendan. "Positive Emotions: The Emerging Science of Feelings." *Institute of Noetic Sciences Newsletter,* 12 (Fall 1984): 5-18.

Rickert, M. Lynn and Koffman, Andrew: "The Use of Groups with Cancer Patients," in *Group Psychotherapy and Counseling,* Milton Seligman (ed.). New York: University Park Press, 1982.

Roraback, Dick. "Cancer Is a Laughing Matter at This Clinic." *Los Angeles Times,* March 12, 1986, sec. 5, p. 1.

Schmale, A. H. and Iker, H. "The Psychological Setting of Uterine Cervical Cancer." *Annals of the New York Academy of Sciences,* 125: 807–813, Jan. 21, 1966.

Siegel, Bernard S. *Love, Medicine & Miracles.* New York: Harper & Row, 1986.

Sime, Wesley E. "Psychological Benefits of Exercise." *Advances,* I (Fall 1984): 15–29.

Simonton, O. Carl; Matthews-Simonton, Stephanie; and Creighton, James L. *Getting Well Again.* Los Angeles: J. P. Tarcher, 1978.

Sklar, L. S. and Anisman, H. "Stress and Cancer." *Psychological Bulletin,* 89: 369–406, May 1981.

Sontag, Susan. *Illness as Metaphor.* New York: Vintage Books, 1977.

Steward, Anita L. *Measuring the Ability to Cope with Serious Illness.* Santa Monica: Rand Corporation, 1983.

"Studies Show Hope Can Play a Role in a Patient's Risk, Illness and Death." *Medical World News,* June 11, 1984, pp. 101–102.

Videka, L. M. "Psychosocial Adaptations in a Medical Self-Help Group," in *Self-Help Groups for Coping with Crisis,* M. L. Lieberman, L. D. Borman and Associates (eds.). San Francisco: Jossey-Bass, 1979.

Walshe, Walter H. *Nature and Treatment of Cancer.* London: Taylor and Walton, 1846.

Wellisch, David K. and Yager, Joel. "Is There a Cancer-Prone Personality?" *Ca,* 33 (May/June 1983): 145–153.

Wortman, C. B. and Dunkel-Schetter, C. "Interpersonal Relationships and Cancer." *Journal of Social Issues,* 35: 120–155, Winter 1979.

Yalom, Irving, "Exploring Group Work Concepts: Similarities and Differences," in *Cancer and The Group Experience.* Los Angeles: American Cancer Society, 1976,

INDEX